PHYSICIAN ALIGNMENT

Ensuring Success with Negotiations, Payment Systems, and Education of Stakeholders

American Association for PHYSICIAN LEADERSHIP

Max Reiboldt, CPA
COKER GROUP

978-0-9907241-3-1 Print
978-0-9907241-4-8 eBook
Published by **American Association for Physician Leadership, Inc.**
PO Box 96503 | BMB 97493 | Washington, DC 20090-6503

Website: www.physicianleaders.org

13 8 7 6 5 4 3 2 1

Copyedited, typeset, indexed, and printed in the United States of America

PUBLISHER
Nancy Collins

EDITORIAL ASSISTANT
Jennifer Weiss

DESIGN & LAYOUT
Carter Publishing Studio

COPYEDITOR
Pat George

Table of Contents

ABOUT THE AUTHOR

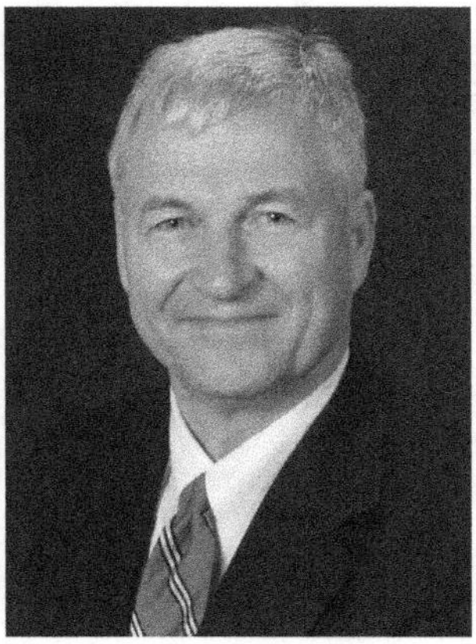

Max Reiboldt, president and CEO of Coker Group, has over 40 years of total experience primarily focused on healthcare. Mr. Reiboldt provides sound tactical and strategic solutions to hospitals, medical practices, health systems, and other healthcare entities through keen analysis and problem solving. Working with organizations of all sizes, he engages in consulting projects with organizations nationwide. His expertise encompasses physician–hospital alignment initiatives, hospital service line development, clinical integration initiatives, financial analyses, mergers and acquisitions, hospital and practice strategic planning, ancillary services development, PHO/IPA/MSO development, practice appraisals, and accountable care era consultation. As the industry adapts to many changes in response to healthcare reform, Mr. Reiboldt is providing hands-on consultation to hospitals, health systems, and large practices.

Reiboldt has led Coker's growth since 1996 to its position today as one of the leading healthcare consulting firms in the United States and abroad. He is an accomplished public speaker on healthcare management topics and has authored or contributed to many of Coker Group's 60-plus books. Recent titles include *Relative Value Units in the Medical Practice, Second Edition* (©2014 Greenbranch Publishing) and *The Healthcare Executive's Guide to Physician-Hospital Alignment* (©2013, Health Leaders Media).

A graduate of Harding University, Reiboldt is a licensed certified public accountant in Georgia and Louisiana, and a member of the American Institute of Certified Public Accountants, Healthcare Financial Management Association, and American Society of Appraisers, Mr. Reiboldt is also a member of the American College of Healthcare Executives.

ABOUT THE CONTRIBUTORS

FRANK ALLEN

Frank Allen is a senior associate with Coker Group and has more than 20 years of experience in financial services. Mr. Allen has specialized experience in hospital/physician alignment, healthcare valuations, compensation reviews, financial modeling, fairness/FMV opinions, and financial analyses specifically for Coker's financial advisory services and alignment teams. He has extensive experience in process improvement, financial reporting, and budgeting with prior experience that includes P&L responsibility for national and international companies with multi-site divisions and gross revenues of more than $250 million and budget tracking responsibility up to $1.2 billion. He holds a BBA in accounting from Harding University.

JUSTIN CHAMBLEE, MACC, CPA

As a vice president at Coker Group, Justin Chamblee works with clients in a variety of strategic and financial areas, mainly dealing with physician compensation and hospital-physician transactions. Projects include developing and redesigning physician compensation plans for private practices and hospital-employed settings, as well as providing guidance to hospitals, physicians, and legal counsel as to the appropriateness of transactions between a hospital and a physician. He frequently speaks on healthcare conference faculties and has authored several books in cooperation with publishers such as Greenbranch Publishing, American Medical Association, and HealthLeaders Media. Prior to joining Coker Group, Mr. Chamblee worked for PricewaterhouseCoopers in their audit practice. He has a BBA in accounting and a master's of accounting from Abilene Christian University. He is licensed as a Certified Public Accountant in Texas and is a member of the American Institute of Certified Public Accountants.

JESSICA COMBS

As a staff associate in Coker Group's Financial Advisory Alignment Services division, Jessica Combs engages in consulting projects with physicians and health systems nationwide. Her career in the healthcare consulting field started in 2008 when she joined Coker Group to assist in the Community Needs Assessment (CNA) research and development process. She ensures accurate and realistic reporting, and is responsible for the initial development of the CNA report and recommendations based on the statistical data available. After several years of working in this capacity, Ms. Combs transitioned to her role in financial advisory services, where she engages in various due diligence reviews, compensation model development, and market research for tangible asset valuations. She has a BS in space physics from Embry-Riddle Aeronautical University. Her scientific background allows her to think critically and strategically, while assisting in the myriad assignments Coker entrusts to her.

AIMEE GREETER, MPH

Aimee Greeter is a vice president at Coker Group with specialized experience in alignment, strategic planning, accountable care responsiveness, compensation, mergers and collaborations, operational issues, and financial management. Ms. Greeter focuses on working with nonprofit and for-profit hospitals and health systems of all sizes, and larger single and multi-specialty physician practices. A popular program speaker, she is frequently engaged by highly respected organizations across the nation. Her accomplishments include the authorship of numerous articles and books. Ms. Greeter attained a BS with honors in human biology from Michigan State University and an MPH in health policy and management from The Rollins School of Public Health at Emory University.

CRAIG HUNTER

Serving as Coker Group's business development leader, Craig Hunter is a senior vice president. He works with health systems, hospital-based networks, multi- and single-specialty groups, and independent physician practices facilitating phases of integration and alignment and practice development, including mergers, strategic planning, management reviews, and negotiations. Mr. Hunter speaks frequently to health system and physician executives, administrators, and other healthcare professionals, and is a published author on practice management topics such as compensation, integration, and physician recruitment and employment.

MADIHA KHAN, MPH

Madiha Khan, staff associate for Coker Group's Financial Advisory and Alignment Services (FAAS) division, works with the FAAS team on strategic planning, accountable care responsiveness, and compensation projects. Her experience also includes presentation development for Coker's various speaking engagements and webinars, and the co-authorship of a variety of healthcare articles and publications. Ms. Khan is a graduate of the University of Virginia with a BA in psychology and minor in biology. She received an MPH in health policy and management from the Rollins School of Public Health at Emory University.

ELLIS M. "MAC" KNIGHT, MD

Ellis "Mac" Knight is senior vice president and chief medical officer of Coker Group, where he oversees Coker's hospital operations and strategic services division. In addition, he has led the development of GlidePath Health, a comprehensive suite of services designed to operationalize clinically integrated organizations such as ACOs. He continues to practice as an internist/hospitalist on a part-time basis.

Prior to joining Coker, Dr. Knight served in a variety of roles at Palmetto Health in Columbia, South Carolina. After 12 years in private medical practice, he started the first hospital medicine group in South Carolina. He helped to grow and manage Palmetto Health's more than 200 employed physicians. He served as the senior vice president of ambulatory services with responsibility for all outpatient activities at this three-hospital system. In 2009, he led the development of and served as the executive medical director for the Palmetto Health Quality Collaborative, Palmetto Health's unique and very successful clinical integration program.

Dr. Knight graduated from Stanford University with a BA degree in human biology. He received his medical degree, with honors, from the University of Oregon Health Science Center's School of Medicine and earned an MBA from the University of Massachusetts at Amherst. He holds a clinical faculty appointment, as an associate professor of medicine, with the University of South Carolina School of Medicine and is a fellow of the American College of Physicians, American College of Healthcare Executives, and the Society of Hospital Medicine.

ERICA LINDQUIST

Erica Lindquist is a staff associate for Coker Group's Financial Advisory and Alignment Services division. Ms. Lindquist provides consulting services on compensation review and model development, fair market value (FMV) opinions, and hospital/physician alignment. She also assists in presentation research and development for Coker's various speaking engagements. Ms. Lindquist is a graduate of Berry College with a BS in psychology and a minor in business. She received a master of business administration from the Coles College of Business at Kennesaw State University.

MARK REIBOLDT

Mark Reiboldt, vice president of Coker Group, provides counsel on strategy and financial consulting engagements for healthcare organizations across the nation. His experience as a financial analyst in the financial services and communication sectors has included engagements involving multi-billion dollar transactions. Mr. Reiboldt serves on the boards of numerous for-profit and not-for-profit organizations within healthcare and other arenas. He received a BA in political science from Georgia State University and an MSc in financial economics from the University of London.

ABOUT COKER GROUP

Coker Group is a national healthcare advisory firm that works with hospitals and physician groups to develop customized solutions that have an impact on your bottom line. Our advisors have the experience and creativity to find the right solution for you and your market. We have sat on both sides of the table for more than three decades—and we know that every situation has unique characteristics. Hospitals and physician practices are both struggling to do more with less. Our clients trust our understanding of the business of healthcare and find our advice leads to real financial and operational impact.

With the rapid changes in healthcare, there are no cookie-cutter solutions that work. Our experienced advisors start by observing and listening to you and your unique circumstances in order to hand-craft a solution that is right for you.

We believe in showing our clients the most valuable part of our work—the thinking behind our recommendations—rather than hiding behind a black box. We'll walk you through the thought process that led to our plan of action, so you know the Why and not just the How of what we are advising.

At Coker Group, we are more than consultants. We take ownership of your challenges, roll up our sleeves, and get in the trenches with you to solve problems.

ACKNOWLEDGEMENTS

We extend our sincere thanks to Nancy Collins and Greenbranch Publishing for their continued confidence and ongoing participation with us to inform and educate the many participants in the healthcare arena through various venues. Knowledge of and advice in the business of healthcare is the greatest gift we can share with hospital executives and physicians; experience is often the best teacher.

Also, we are grateful for our many clients over the years and the lessons we have learned from the experience of engaging with them. Working with our clients through the challenges and changes they encounter has benefited us as individuals and as an organization. We hope that we have helped every client to achieve their goals and to improve their positions.

Thank you to all.

Foreword

In light of the evolution of healthcare, physician alignment is a legitimate issue for providers who now function in the era of accountable care. The dilemmas providers face are less about whether to align with other entities and more about how to ensure success. Many options are available. The key issue is how to arrive in the best situation possible.

To prepare, participants must stay informed, stay flexible, be realistic, and prepare in advance for changes that are certain to occur over the duration of the arrangement. Possibly the most volatile area is the need for appropriate compensation. The most vital area, perhaps, is the call for physician leadership.

The chapters that follow address the challenges of ensuring successful physician alignment. The purpose in writing them is to help readers to:

- Understand the different alignment options available to practitioners;
- Learn how each of the alignment options fits in with the future of healthcare, including ACOs and risk-based payer contracts;
- Recognize the benefits and challenges of physician alignment outside of a hospital relationship;
- Identify the critical success factors in an alignment model;
- Develop strategies related to creating a new alignment relationship with other physicians or investors; and
- Educate the key stakeholders on how to be involved in the process from concept to implementation and beyond.

The options that are available continue to attest that no one model of alignment fits every scenario, specialty, or marketplace. The challenges and pitfalls are predictable. The resources in this book identify a clear pathway to ensuring success with negotiations, payment systems, and education of stakeholders.

CHAPTER 1

The Healthcare Industry Today: Changes and Challenges

Healthcare in America is ever dynamic. Those who have experienced the healthcare delivery system first-hand—as a provider, patient, business advisor, legal counsel, or a combination—have seen unparalleled changes in recent years. As we dig deeply into the key drivers of these changes, we will begin with the basics of the changes and challenges that are transpiring—changes and challenges that may never abate as our American society continues to evolve.

Our primary focus is from the perspective of healthcare providers: physicians, hospitals, allied healthcare providers, ancillary provider services, etc. These individuals and entities, fully dedicated to the provision of healthcare with utmost quality and professionalism, are being asked to continue to provide quality service despite extensive changes in structure and reimbursement. We will review the details in the context of current and impending changes.

So, let's consider specific issues healthcare provides are confronting today and those we anticipate they will face in the near future.

STRUCTURE OF DELIVERY OF HEALTHCARE SERVICES

Traditionally, healthcare providers in the United States are autonomous in their delivery of care. While they may coordinate and communicate with other providers to some extent, they tend to keep others at arm's length for the protection and privacy of the patient, and to maintain independence among various provider disciplines. One of the major changes and challenges confronting the healthcare industry today is the structure of the delivery of services, because the emphasis now is on *coordination of care* among providers. Providers must exchange extensive information and data, including outcomes. No longer will physicians limit their information sharing with other providers to an "available upon request" basis.

All clinical information pertaining to a patient must be available across provider disciplines. The providers may all be part of a single integrated delivery system or, if they maintain legal separation, will form entities that allow for exchange of information. The most prominent type of entity to effectuate these structures is the *clinically integrated network (CIN),* also referred to as a *clinically integrated organization (CIO).* Another version is the *accountable care organization (ACO).* These consortiums may comprise the same legal entities or they may work together on a contractual basis, but their structure and the delivery of services will be as one entity.

In exploring the makeup of ACOs, CINs, and CIOs, we will consider not only their goals and objectives, but their formation and daily functionality. These entities exist now, and their numbers are growing rapidly. Within the next five years, operating as CINs and ACOs will be the norm; the delivery of services will be fully coordinated.

Clinical integration enables patients to receive a variety of health services from the same legal or aligned organization or entity, which streamlines administrative processes and increases the potential for the delivery of high-quality healthcare. Although the structure of these entities will not require health systems to employ physicians, physicians can be, and many will be, employees. In the future, physicians must be clinically integrated in every sense of the definition.

Consolidation of providers is a fundamental structure of healthcare delivery. Although consolidation is not new, the ability to maintain such entities will be essential going forward. Consequently, mergers of healthcare systems, physician groups, and other related healthcare providers will continue. Those merged entities will be the consolidated providers, along with those with whom they may contract to form CINs. The number of independent health systems will decrease as more consolidation occurs. Notwithstanding this point, the issues of restrictive trade and anti-trust are a major consideration and in fact many such attempts to consolidate have been challenged and even negated as a result of anti-trust assertions. Nonetheless, the era of healthcare provider consolidation will continue along with the challenges of being in compliance with anti-trust regulations.

We will address to some degree the question of whether a health system, even a community hospital, can remain independent through the next wave of healthcare provider structures.

So what are the main drivers of this new delivery structure, especially for healthcare providers who are looking to consolidate? They are:

1. **Market position preservation/improvement.** Although the industry is concerned about the good of the patient, healthcare is a business, regardless of whether the entity is for-profit or not-for-profit. The ability to maintain and grow market share through the new delivery structure and consolidation is essential.
2. **Care coordination improvement.** The capability to coordinate care among a cross-section of providers is a "win-win" arrangement for all, including the new system of healthcare providers. Communication through clinically integrated structures will improve the efficiency and quality of care—an issue we explore throughout the book.
3. **Cost reductions and efficiency improvements.** The focus of this driver is the reduction of needless procedures, tests, and overall inefficiencies that come with a lack of coordination and communication. Eliminating wastes and inefficiencies will enhance the healthcare delivery system structure; providers can achieve many of these improvements through consolidation.
4. **Standardization of clinical protocols.** Communication and care coordination will help establish standards that will allow clear clinical pathways to be streamlined, thorough, and efficient. Most healthcare providers and payers would prefer standard-

ization of clinical protocols. Discussions of payer and reimbursement systems occur in this context.

5. **Exception reductions.** Although exceptions to clinical protocols and some unique situations will occur, the standardization, care coordination, and overall improved efficiencies will reduce the variances that happen far too frequently.
6. **Quality enhancement.** The ability to maintain high levels of clinical quality outcomes through better definition, measurement, and analytics will prove invaluable during the establishment of new consolidated healthcare provider structures. These elements enhance care and provide better patient satisfaction and appreciation of the services.
7. **Utilization (over-utilization) management.** While some would argue that most healthcare provider diagnostic and operative procedures are necessary within our present system, a lot of second guessing can occur, even after the fact. Coordination of care will address this matter, driving down costs and focusing reimbursement in the appropriate areas.

The structural changes for the delivery of healthcare services will require that a variety of healthcare providers make tactical, strategic, transformational adjustments. The mere fact that previously disparate groups will come together to address the following topics suggests substantial challenges:

- Structure and governance;
- Infrastructure and funding;
- Participation criteria;
- Performance objectives;
- Leadership among physicians;
- Information technology;
- Funds allocation; and
- Contracting with payers.

As key components of the CIN, these elements present major challenges in a traditional setting; they present even more stress in the new structures of delivery.

So why are markets moving to new structures of delivery of services? We explore these issues in the remainder of this chapter and throughout the book. The tactical, strategic, and transformational drivers of these evolving structures often are implemented through various specific entities, as we illustrate in Figure 1-1.

As we continue to explore provider alignment and the various supporting models, we will consider how they work and their place within the continuum of the healthcare industry today and in the future.

DRIVING FORCES FOR CHANGE: REIMBURSEMENT PARADIGM SHIFTS

Figure 1-2 illustrates the driving forces for change within our healthcare industry specifically related to a shifting paradigm for the traditional healthcare delivery model versus that of the accountable care era model. Chiefly related to these changing paradigms are the shifts in reimbursement.

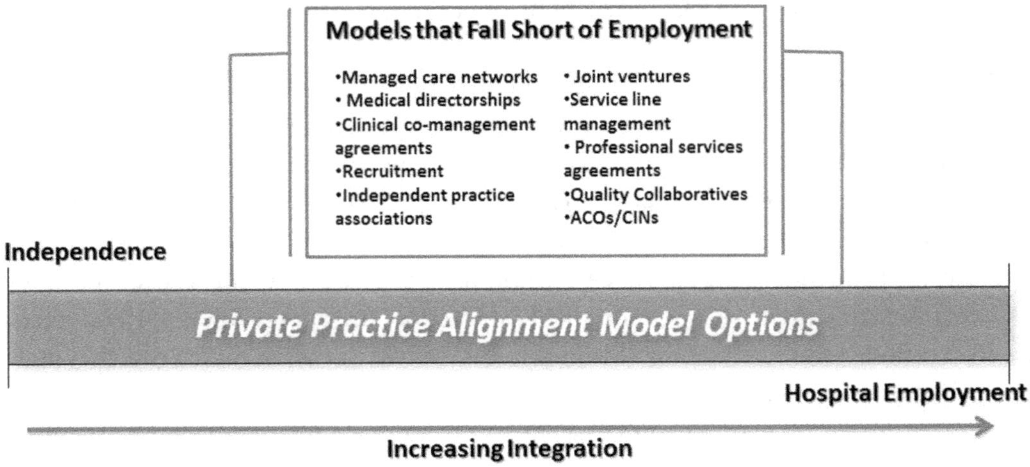

FIGURE 1-1. Alignment Model Spectrum

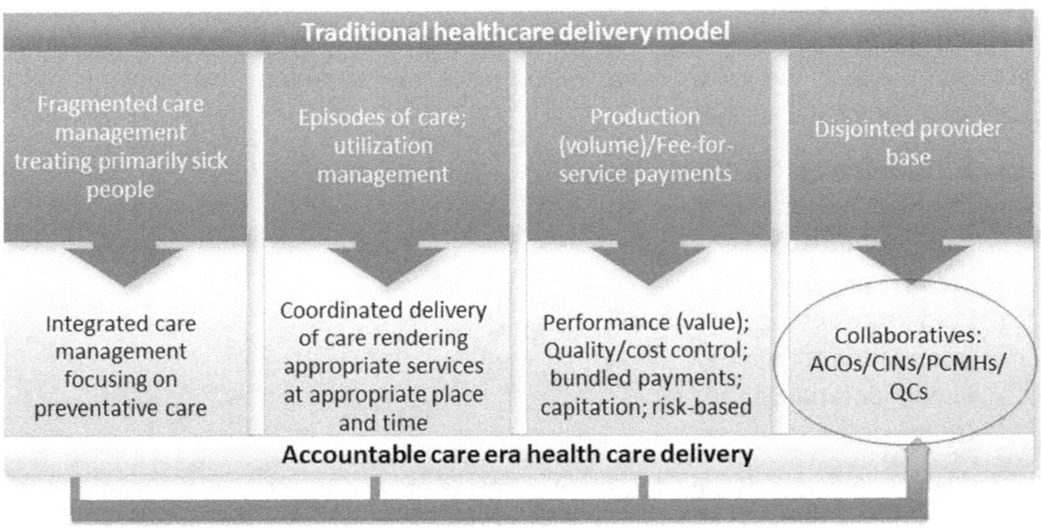

FIGURE 1-2. Driving Forces for Change: Paradigm Shifts

The traditional healthcare delivery model is fragmented, with an emphasis on treating the sickness and the disease and minimal coordination of care. It is characterized by episodic care and attempts to manage utilization. The reimbursement structure, then, is based on volume, with payments for services rendered as opposed to outcomes, quality, or cost savings. As a result, the provider base is disorganized, disjointed, and somewhat dysfunctional.

Conversely, the accountable care-era delivery system considers true integration and care management that focuses on preventing illness as opposed to primarily treating the sick. Accountable care treats illnesses, but the objective is to provide better-managed and coordinated care. Delivery of care is coordinated among the providers from all disciplines and facilities, including hospital, physician, and allied healthcare providers. The reimbursement structure focuses more on value and performance, using quality outcomes and cost controls as the primary determinants.

Coordination of care and the integration of providers results in reimbursement as bundled payments. Forms of capitation and payments that reward for performance yet can also be punitive for lack of performance (i.e., risk based) are possible. As for the provider base, collaboratives are the norm via the various forms of consolidation discussed earlier in the chapter. The standard way to provide care is through ACOs, CINs, patient-centered medical homes (PCMHs), and quality collaboratives. Here, providers are organized, integrated, and consolidated in their delivery of care.

Reimbursement payments and structures are also changing, as Figure 1-3 illustrates.

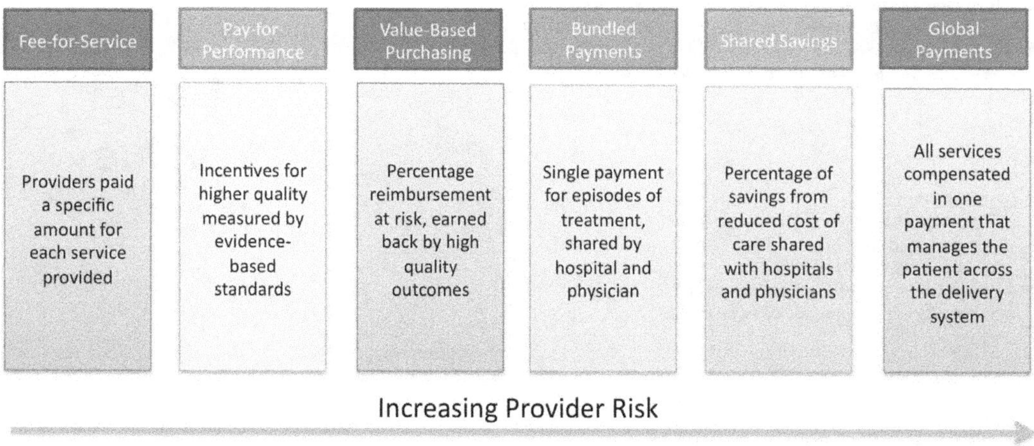

FIGURE 1-3. Driving Forces for Change: Evolving Payment Models

The traditional fee-for-service structure, where providers are paid a specific amount as they render services (and for the volume), still exists. However, the model is changing rapidly. The trend is to move away from fee-for-service and fee-for-volume to pay-for-performance, thus increasing provider risk. This model that incorporates incentives for higher quality measured by evidence-based standards is not new, but it will continue to grow. The prevalence of value-based purchasing, where reimbursement is at risk but is earned back by high-quality outcomes, will increase as well.

With the establishment of CINs and more fully integrated and care-coordinated structures, bundled payments will become the reimbursement norm. Single payments for episodes of treatment, shared by a cross-section of providers from hospitals to physicians and others, will become the dominant payment model. Shared savings programs are being established in many areas that have certain specialties and specific procedures (often surgical procedures). Here, providers share in savings when they are able to validate a reduced cost of care. The global payment method of reimbursement, where the percentage of the savings from the overall reduced cost of managing populations, will rise in prominence, especially within CINs, as they mature.

The reimbursement vehicles of the new payment paradigm will range from fee-for-service to global payments, and various models between the extremes. The payment variance means that providers must be organized and coordinated in their care to realize maximum payment for their services. Wringing out costs within our healthcare system is at the core of these new structures and is an issue everyone must address. Quality enhancements through good outcomes are also important, always aiming for achievement of high value coupled with cost reductions. Figure 1-4 illustrates how this all culminates to value.

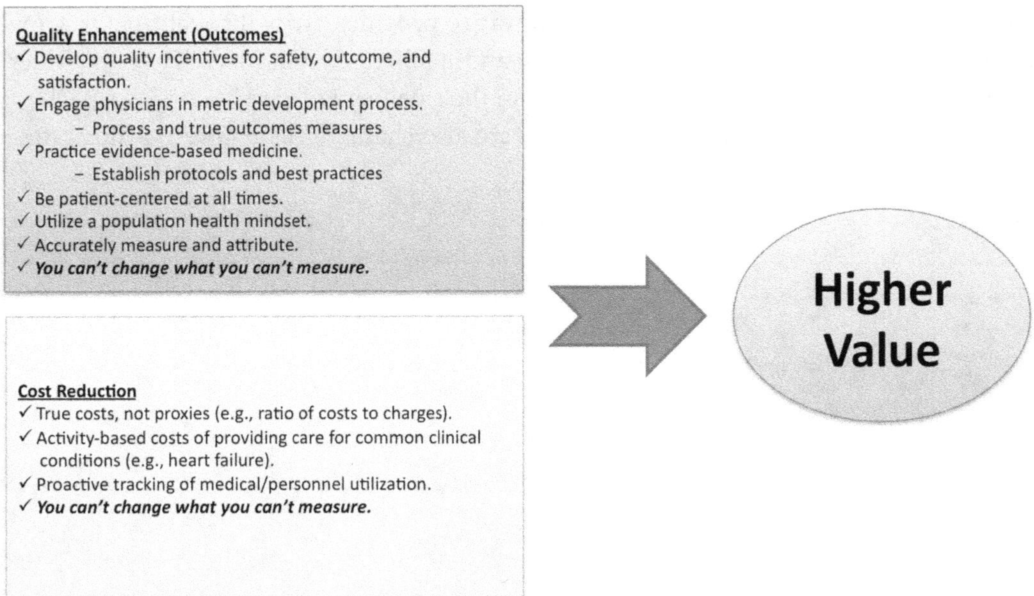

FIGURE 1-4. It *All* Culminates to Value

The ultimate challenge for providers will be to provide high-quality healthcare through a cost-efficient clinical delivery system. The requirement will mean managing large blocks of the population to deliver value through better outcomes at lower cost—with limited funds!

ALIGNMENT OF PROVIDERS

As healthcare systems and physicians realize the requirements of the accountable care era, they understand that the changes and challenges call for cooperation and alignment. All providers must have a common purpose and develop seamless working relationships relative to business and clinical-care coordination.

Realizing the goals and objectives of the accountable care structure, where quality, safety, and cost efficiencies are the key to success, requires the application of these six overarching principles:

1. **Common purpose.** Health systems, physicians, and all providers must understand that the demand is for improved patient outcomes, reduced inefficiencies and waste, and controlled costs. In this context, providers must understand the aligned organizations' "Newco" culture while minding relevant legal/regulatory requirements and barriers.
2. **Common values and goals/objectives.** Alignment means that all providers work as partners; one is not an employee or customer of the other. As partners, they should

work together to benefit the entire organization and to maintain their individual responsibilities for quality.

3. **Defined structure.** The good of the whole should be an overarching principle at all times with few, if any individual "carve outs." Leaders should function as leaders, managing projects and overseeing the "big picture" requirements, but they should also be inclusive of their colleagues' input and overall contributions. Education and information exchange are essential among the aligned partners. Leaders should identify and address—or dismiss—any "slackers" or naysayers within the organization.
4. **Standardized improvement methods.** Standardization is essential to cost effectiveness, elimination of waste, and overall efficiency. Simplicity is also important and may entail eliminating complex processes and concepts that overlap among the aligned partners.
5. **Resourceful nature.** Resourcefulness is not easy, but it is essential. For many, it will require adjustment and adaptation.
6. **Engaging style.** At the end of this process, no single entity—whether it be the health system, CIN, or another organization—can be fully in control. Everyone must be engaged and aligned. Involving physicians from the outset is essential. Identifying leaders is likewise critical. Everyone should adapt and realize that this is the new way of delivering healthcare and, as such, is the economic model that will become the norm. Disjointed and dysfunctional coordination of care cannot exist in this "new world."

Based on these tenets, the definition of various alignment models among physicians and health systems (and among physicians and other physicians) is important and yet not necessarily mutually exclusive. Figure 1-5 illustrates the typical alignment models, defined from limited to moderate to full.

The need to align is clear and the models can vary, meaning that some limited forms can be mixed with moderate and fuller forms of alignment. Ultimately, capturing and addressing a large population's health management will call for fuller forms of alignment (full integration). A CIN or ACO will be the most likely to surface as the most suitable models. The specific alignment models will be addressed in greater depth in subsequent chapters.

COSTS AND QUALITY

The concept of lowering costs while maintaining quality is fundamental to the new era of accountable care and will become more visible in the reimbursement models that exist under such a structure. Lower cost and high quality will require *tactical*, *strategic*, and *transformational* processes. Physicians and hospitals will have to align and adapt to the key tenets of such alignment models to achieve the best efficiencies of costs and quality of care. Payers and patients will demand no less, nor should they.

Knowing one's costs will be critically important; being able to measure them will be essential. Quality, while nebulous, is also an essential element of any new era structure, and is being calculated more frequently. Performance improvement and quality can be demonstrated through the following:

- **Variance in cost reduction.** Minimize variable physician performance, not related to patient disease/illness traits.

Limited Integration	Moderate Integration	Full Integration
▪ (P2P) **Managed Care Networks (Independent Practice Associations, Physician Hospital Organizations):** Loose alliances for contracting purposes ▪ (P2P) **Recruitment/Incubation:** Economic assistance for new physicians ▪ (P2P) **Group (Legal-Only) Merger:** Unites parties under common legal entity without an operational merger ▪ (P2H) **Call Coverage Stipends:** Pay for unassigned ED call ▪ (P2H) **Medical Directorships:** Specific clinical oversight duties	▪ (P2H) **Service Line Management:** Management of all specialty services within the hospital ▪ (P2H) **MSO/ISO:** Ties hospitals to physician's businesis ▪ (P2H) **Clinical Co-Management:** Physicians become actively engaged in clinical operations and oversight of applicable service line at the hospital ▪ (P2P or P2H) **Equity Group Assimilation:** Ties entities via legal agreement; joint practice ownership ▪ (P2P or P2H) **Joint Ventures:** Unites parties under common enterprise; difficult to structure; legal hurdles	▪ (P2P or P2H) **ACO/CIN/QC:** Participation in an organization focus on improving quality/cost of care for government or non-governmental payers; may be driven by practices or hospital groups ▪ (P2H) **Employment:** Strongest alignment; minimizes economic risk for physicians ▪ (P2P) **Group (Legal and Operational Merger):** Unites parties under common legal entity with full integration of operations

P2P—Typical Physician-to-Physician

P2H—Typical Physician-to-Hospital

P2P or P2H—Either Physician-Physician or Physician-Hospital

FIGURE 1-5. Traditional Alignment Model Descriptions

- **Unnecessary care reduction.** Reduce avoidable, less than fully productive, and duplicative services.
- **Clinical restructuring.** Assure optimal treatment in the best and most appropriate setting and provider structure.
- **System optimization.** Supply care where best suited, whether it be preventative, primary care, upstream, or a combination. Overall, manage population health. Examples include minimizing supply chain cost; optimizing staffing and productivity; reducing length of stay and readmissions; and facilitating early step down to the appropriate service entity. Additional elements include partnering with local retail clinics and offering the appropriate level of non-urgent care; engaging disease-based medical homes; and supporting patient engagement, including use of electronic mail and telehealth.

CONCLUSION

The standards for the healthcare industry will continue to change at a relatively rapid pace, creating more challenges and changing structures for all healthcare providers. As we continue to explore these varied structures, relationships, and strategies going forward, we will provide more insights as to how best to approach and deal with these dramatic and dynamic situations.

CHAPTER 2

Options for Contemporary Alignment

Traditional alignment models, such as professional services agreements, clinical co-management agreements, and employment, although still relevant today, have begun sharing the stage with more "progressive" alignment strategies. These models oftentimes build upon the foundation created by traditional alignment models and typically incorporate significant aspects of clinical integration. Commonly known as accountable care organizations (ACOs), clinically integrated networks/organizations (CINs/CIOs), quality collaboratives (QCs), and patient-centered medical homes (PCMHs), these contemporary alignment strategies, regardless of the acronym, are fundamentally similar in nature and function. In this chapter, we explain the options available to providers in the realm of contemporary alignment and discuss the main considerations for effectuating these strategies.

ALIGNMENT AS STAGE ONE, AND INTEGRATION AS STAGE TWO

As providers find themselves in the midst of the accountable care era, looking around anxiously for the appropriate way to respond to ensure their ongoing success, it is important that they consider a strategic response that incorporates elements of both traditional and contemporary alignment. In fact, a successful accountable care era strategy involves traditional alignment as stage one, and clinical integration (or contemporary alignment) as stage two. This two-stage approach allows organizations to move gradually toward an operational *system* that is sustainable, engages all parties involved, and, above all, is value- and patient-centric.

Forming a clinically integrated/accountable care organization requires significant collaboration among many different stakeholders, and often among competitors. A go-forward traditional alignment strategy is the best way to ensure successful integration for such collaborative models, particularly between distinct private groups. Through the use of professional service agreements (PSAs), medical directorships, service line management agreements, etc., healthcare entities are able to lay the groundwork to move their partners toward the cultural shift that is occurring within healthcare.

More specifically, traditional alignment models are designed to accomplish several goals, including the following, which are all precursors to contemporary alignment:

- Foster an organizational culture that supports teamwork;

- Promote an attitude for success and remain positive, especially considering the uncertainties and flexibility requested; and
- Alleviate many of the risks and challenges often associated with ACO/CIN development by building the elements of collaboration and care coordination.

Without sufficient alignment and harmony between disparate groups of providers, the quality of patient care, as well as population health management functions, are likely to suffer. Simply put, while contemporary alignment in the form of clinical integration and care delivery transformation are the ultimate goals, initial traditional alignment is its primary vehicle.

CONTEMPORARY ALIGNMENT MODELS: THE BASICS

Within the current healthcare market, the number of contemporary alignment structures is increasing rapidly. As reported by Premier, Inc.'s 2013 survey of more than 100 healthcare executives, provider participation in an ACO model has nearly quadrupled since spring 2012, when the ACO participation rate was approximately 4.8%. These rates are projected to continue to rise, with participation projected to double by the end of 2014 to 50%.[1] As the reimbursement paradigm continues to shift from being strictly fee-for-volume to also including fee-for-value payments, this trend is likely to continue and be emblematic for all four contemporary alignment options available today: ACOs, CINs, QCs, and PCMHs.

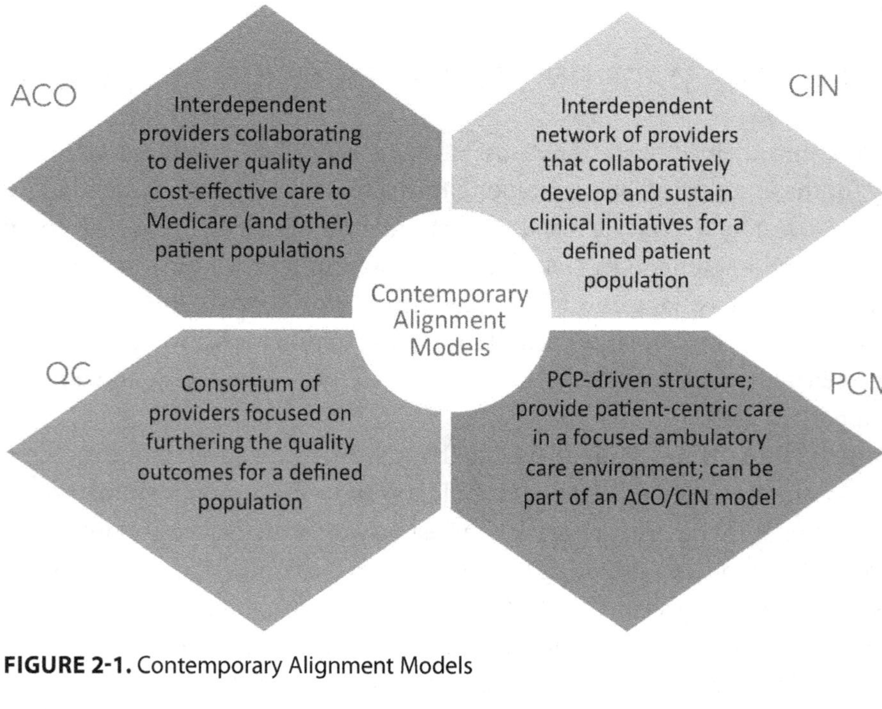

FIGURE 2-1. Contemporary Alignment Models

As illustrated by Figure 2-1, the four models are very similar conceptually. They all represent risk-based, clinically integrated entities that are bound by the same cultural ties and function along one common information technology platform such that data can easily be shared among each party for the delivery of *valuable* care to its respective patient population. Each model is also guided by the Institute of Healthcare's Triple Aim, which is an approach for optimizing health system performance by:

- Improving the patient experience of care (including quality and satisfaction);
- Reducing the per-capita cost of healthcare; and
- Improving the health of populations.

The first two points of the Triple Aim outline the value proposition (defined as "outcome per unit of cost") while the third describes population health management. As such, all contemporary alignment models exist to advance the value proposition. Despite these similarities, none of these models works as "one size fits all"; several factors dictate which model is the most appropriate for the provider group. In some cases, a contemporary alignment model may not be necessary at all. For example, if a provider's current market is projected to remain strictly fee-for-service (FFS) for some time, there is little *immediate* need to pursue contemporary alignment. We note, however, that the move toward fee-for-value (FFV) payments is a nationwide trend, although some areas are realizing this shift at a faster rate than others.

OPTIONS FOR STRUCTURING A CONTEMPORARY ALIGNMENT MODEL

Single- or Multi-Specialty Models

Must contemporary alignment structures *always* be multi-specialty in nature? It depends on several factors. For many reasons, single-specialty partnerships may be easier to effectuate than multi-specialty ones and, thus, some constituencies (including well-established single-specialty private practices) may prefer single-specialty clinically integrated models. This concept is becoming increasingly common. For example, US Oncology announced its decision to explore a Medicare ACO specifically focused on oncology. However, single-specialty ACOs/CINs/QCs must focus on the care of patient *populations,* and, thereby, these organizations must be multi-specialty in function to meet their patients' needs. While single-specialty models are possible, they must incorporate methodologies for coordinating care with varied specialties of providers, several other single-specialty ACOs, or multi-specialty ACOs in their market to achieve the Triple Aim.

Physician-Based Options

Contemporary alignment does not necessarily entail robust relationships with hospital providers. Physician-based models are gaining momentum in the industry as private physicians continue to explore long-term strategies that do not require complete loss of independence and autonomy—a factor that many providers associate with hospital relationships. In this scenario, ACOs, CINs, and QCs are established under the control and direction of a network of aligned private practices/physicians who have joined forces to finance and effectuate these undertakings. Arguably, these providers are more entrepreneurial-minded and receptive to some element of risk, as they opt to use the current challenges affecting private practices as an opportunity to improve patient care and the practice environment for themselves.

Three notable forms of physician-consolidated structures exist, with two serving as a precursor to a full-form clinically integrated entity: independent practice associations (IPAs) and physician hospital organizations (PHOs). Both of these structures are moderately integrated forms of traditional alignment wherein private physicians have loosely affiliated contractual relationships with each other. For the most part, each practice retains its current status, structure, and operations; however, each physician becomes a part of a separate entity (the IPA/PHO) that affords each group the ability to reap the benefits of a much larger group.

Typically, IPAs/PHOs as a group can contract to provide services to payers and managed-care organizations or enforce group purchasing power. For example, a managed-care plan such as an HMO can negotiate and contract with an IPA, which would then contract with its independent physicians using the negotiated/discounted fees or on a capitation basis. IPAs and PHOs also can contract with hospital systems and ACOs/CINs to provide services. Clearly, under the PHO model (as its name would imply), it is more common for hospitals to be part of the organization as well.

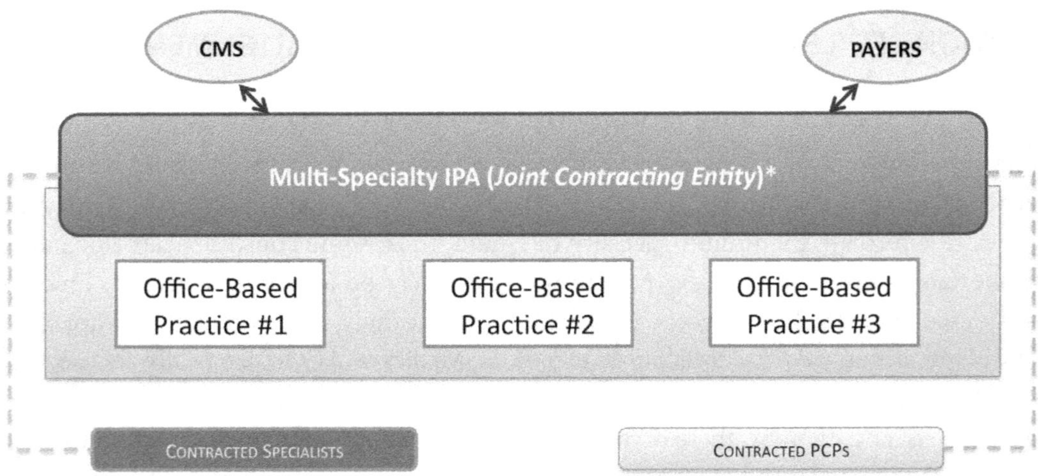

**Can consist of as many private practices as desired by the participating parties.*

FIGURE 2-2. The IPA Model

The mid- to late-1990s saw an abundance of IPAs and PHOs across the country, but many of these organizations were terminated or went dormant due to lack of funding, limited benefits to participants (either real or perceived), or conversion into other forms of alignment. However, more recently, IPAs and PHOs are being resurrected to serve as foundational models for physician-based consortiums such as QCs and CINs. They can provide a forum for their members to improve collective results in case management and manage the quality and cost of patient care. They also can facilitate data collection, analysis, and application of same for the continuous improvement of care-related and operational protocols. Simply put, IPAs give groups of like-minded private physicians the capacity to:

- Design highly reliable, cost-efficient, evidence-based, patient-centric processes of care;
- Develop measurement systems to monitor above processes of care [true outcomes and true costs (i.e., value)];
- Utilize data metrics to drive continuous value improvement and create a true learning organization;
- Create a self-governing system of accountability that holds all participants to the physician-determined standards of care; and
- Apply care processes to drive pricing that will accurately reflect true costs of care delivery.

For most of the aforementioned goals/functions to materialize, all members of the IPA/PHO must be on one electronic health record (EHR) system or use an interface that robustly links the varied systems. After they meet the EHR requirements and the other criteria of clinical integration, and after regulatory bodies officially recognize the entity as a CIN, the organization will be able to enter into direct negotiations with payers for pay-for-performance or value-based contracts. Figure 2-3 illustrates the "look" of such an entity. Depending on the sponsoring payer, this model may be a QC/CIN or an ACO.

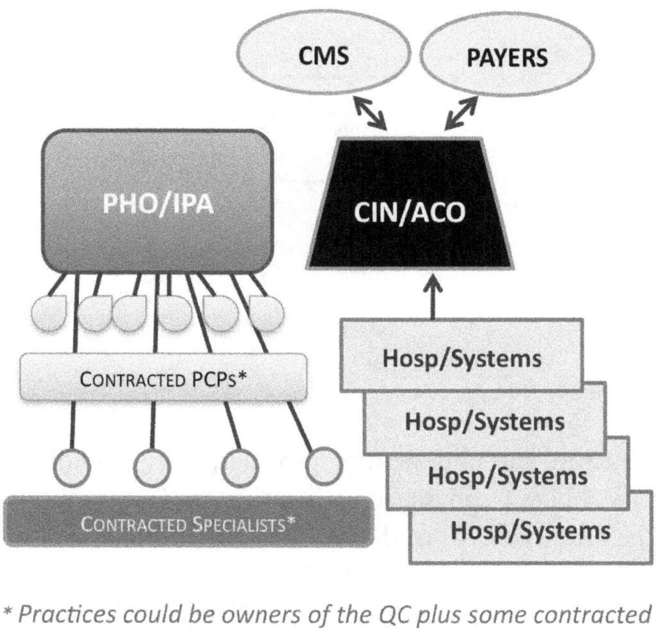

FIGURE 2-3. IPA/PHO-Based Collaborative Structure

Hospital-Based Options

As Figure 2-3 depicts, physician-based collaborative structures should incorporate hospital partners in some manner, even if the incorporation is limited to the physicians continuing to practice in a hospital when patient care necessitates such, and hopefully, engaging that hospital in discussions regarding value creation (referenced above). In fact, a large component of long-term success for providers (both hospitals and private physicians alike) will be driven by their partnerships/ability to work with each other. Nonetheless, hospitals are arguably facing the pressures of change much more than private physicians and, thus, many have been compelled to strategize and reform their current care delivery structures faster than independent providers. Hospitals also have the wherewithal and management expertise necessary to contemplate and, eventually, effectuate an ACO/CIN strategy. Thus, far more hospital-based ACOs/CINs exist than physician-based models at this time.

Drivers of hospital-based collaboratives are the hospital or health system's physicians and administrators who often belong to the governing board and at least one of its sub-committees. Examples of sub-committees include, but are not limited, to:

- Information technology committee;
- Clinical performance/quality committee; and
- Finance/capitalization/compensation committee.

Figure 2-4 depicts the typical hospital-based CIN structure.

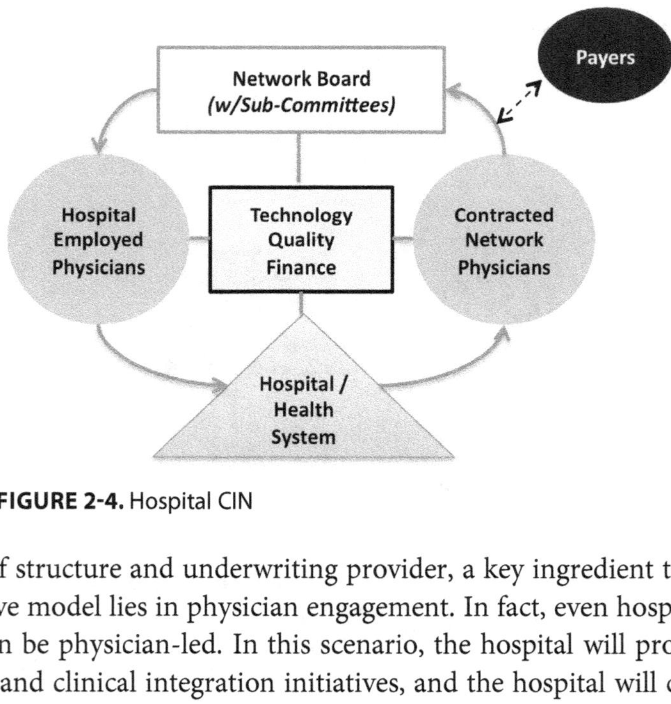

FIGURE 2-4. Hospital CIN

Regardless of structure and underwriting provider, a key ingredient to the success of any collaborative model lies in physician engagement. In fact, even hospital-based QCs/CINs/ACOs can be physician-led. In this scenario, the hospital will provide capital for developmental and clinical integration initiatives, and the hospital will collaborate with the physicians to govern the model on an ongoing basis, to provide continuous feedback regarding the clinical aspects of value-based care, and to maintain open channels of communication. Physicians will be able to oversee day-to-day operations of the CIN, innovate and lead novel clinical integration initiatives and coordinate care, and develop performance measures and metrics that steer the direction of the CIN. However, the hospital will have the final decision-making power on all *major* matters, such as those that involve capital investment.

Physicians form the backbone for all contemporary alignment and are often the driving forces for clinical integration initiatives. As physicians are often considered the drivers of cost, it only makes sense to make them the champions of change. Needless to say, the industry is in the midst of a significant cultural shift. The engagement of physicians will certainly help lead the way to change, as significant clinical buy-in will be necessary for re-tooling a care delivery process. Therefore, physicians arguably are the best-equipped to influence change among support staff, other physicians, non-physician providers, and other caregivers over the entire care delivery continuum. Whether physician-based or hospital-based, new delivery models necessitate *heavy* buy-in from participating providers.

Organizational Options for ACOs/CINs

Providers can organize their clinically integrated business entity in one of several ways:

- Not-for-profit corporation;
- For-profit corporation; or
- Limited liability company (LLC).

Not-for-Profit Corporation

Not-for-profit, tax-exempt ACOs/CINs must have a parent organization that is also tax-exempt per the guidelines of section 501(c)(3) of the Internal Revenue Code. These organizations and their founding hospitals must take several considerations into account; chief among them are legal or regulatory considerations to which only tax-exempt hospitals establishing nonprofit ACOs/CINs are subject.

According to the American Bar Association, tax-exempt hospitals choosing to develop a not-for-profit ACO or CIN should ensure that 1) the clinically integrated entity will advance the hospital's charitable mission and thus, the income generated by the entity can be considered as related business income that will also be tax exempt (the clinically integrated entity can also apply for tax-exempt status independent of the hospital); and 2) ACO/CIN participation does not result in any inurement or impermissible private benefit to the parties involved, which would certainly compromise the organization's tax-exempt status and/or evoke fiscal consequences such as tax penalties.[2]

In general, tax-exempt Medicare Shared Savings Programs (MSSPs) or commercial ACOs will be subject to substantial regulatory scrutiny; thus, it is imperative for these entities to:

- Memorialize the terms of the tax-exempt parent organization's participation in the ACO within a definitive agreement;
- Ensure that the tax-exempt parent organization's portion of any economic benefits realized by the parent organization from the ACO/CIN is equal to its contributions to the ACO/CIN;
- Ensure that the portion of any losses realized by the parent organization from the ACO/CIN is less than its share of benefits; and
- Confirm that all arrangements are within fair market value limitations and compliant with pertinent regulations.

These types of clinically integrated entities are beneficial for providers who want to establish a "progressive" model that is also responsive to the hospital's mission, vision, and purposes. Other benefits include financial transparency, as not-for-profit organizations are expected to report their financial performances routinely.

Nonetheless, several challenges do exist, such as the legal considerations explained above, as well as certain governance and physician engagement concerns. For example, many hospitals serve as the sole corporate member (and thus, the dominant party) of a not-for-profit ACO/CIN model. This type of arrangement can make sufficient physician engagement difficult and may deter certain physicians from being receptive to the idea or model. Fortunately, none of these issues is insurmountable as proven by the number of not-for-profit ACOs currently in existence.

For-Profit Corporation

In a for-profit ACO/CIN model, the parent organization may be for-profit or not-for-profit and the ACO/CIN an incorporated entity with which the parent organization contracts for professional services. Needless to say, the income generated by the ACO/CIN, Inc., will be subject to taxes, although fewer regulatory implications exist in comparison to the not-for-profit model. Oftentimes, the parent organization provides a large portion of the necessary capital to operate the incorporated ACO/CIN entity via preferred stock ownership or loans. The physician members and hospital may hold common stock ownership in equal measures of each other; however, only the parent organization has preferred stock ownership. Any shared savings earned are typically distributed to the participating physicians and the parent organization, although some of these funds may also be used to reinvest in the ACO/CIN, Inc.

This model is attractive for several reasons. For one, both nonprofit and for-profit parent organizations can employ this business structure, and the legal considerations, while still relevant, may not be as burdensome as those associated with obtaining and maintaining tax-exempt status. Further, physician engagement is not necessarily hindered, as the hospital and physicians have relatively the same level of risk and membership; the hospital is able to invest in the entity (disproportionate to the amount of income generated by the entity) through preferred stock ownerships.

Despite these apparent benefits, for-profit hospitals/health systems are wary of ACOs/CINs, citing uncertainty about prospective savings justifying start-up costs as the primary reason. In fact, of the three largest hospital chains, only Tenet Healthcare (the third-largest hospital system) has experimented with ACO-like models. This action includes the development of a commercial ACO in Modesto, California, in January 2012 and the purchase of Vanguard Health Systems in October 2013. Vanguard Health Systems operates the Detroit Medical Center, which is a successful pioneer ACO that realized savings in its first year.

LLC Model

As set forth by the Patient Protection and Affordable Care Act and the MSSP guidelines, ACOs (and CINs) can be separate legal entities or hospital subsidiaries. Under the former scenario, parent organizations generally form the ACO/CIN as an LLC, which is considered under state law to be a separate legal entity from the parent company. The ACO/CIN, LLC, can then independently contract with public and private payers and for the purposes of federal income tax, it will be considered a disregarded entity. This approach is attractive for tax-exempt organizations to establish a not-for-profit clinically integrated entity.

The ACO/CIN, LLC structure has several advantages in that there may be potential tax benefits to participants with limitations on personal risks/liabilities as well as the ability to distribute funds/savings to participating providers. Further, the LLC structure is relatively easy to establish in terms of time and financial resources.

Patient-Centered Medical Home

The PCMH model (Figure 2-5) is arguably the epicenter for all clinically integrated entities. Due to the heavy primary care component that is inherent to the success of all contemporary alignment structures, the medical home model is imperative for effective care coordination and the delivery of preventative medicine within a complete integrated delivery system. Nonetheless, only a quarter of existing private practices represent designated PCMHs per National Committee for Quality Assurance (NCQA) standards. It is likely that this relatively low rate is a result of private practices not being able to make the capital and time investments required to transform their practice into a PCMH.

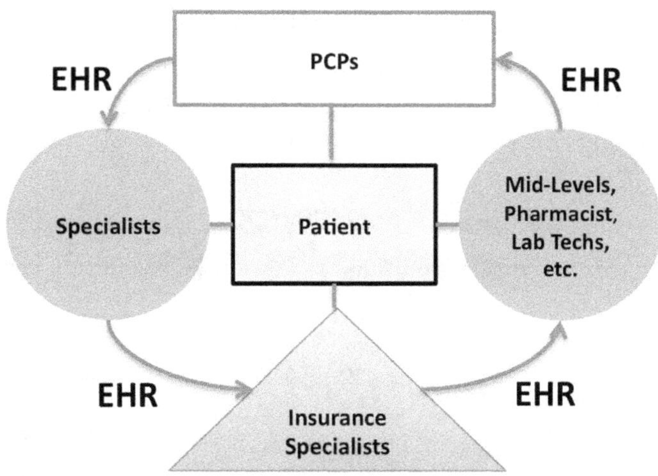

FIGURE 2-5. Typical PCMH Model

We note that the medical home model does not apply only to primary care practices; specialty medical homes, while rare, are also possible. In fact, as of March 2013, the NCQA launched its new designation program specifically targeted toward specialty practices that actively participate in the PCMH model or serve as a medical home "neighbor," called the Patient-Centered Specialty Practice. Ultimately, the specialty practice's decision to pursue the PCMH model is based on the organization's scope of services and patient population composition. A specialty PCMH may be a suitable option for those practices that provide specialty services that have some primary care components (such as those treating chronic disease patients) to a significant portion of their patient population. Alternatively, other specialty services may prefer being a part of the medical home neighborhood wherein they work closely with primary care practices, which serve as the medical home's center.

Unlike ACOs and CINs, which generally entail the development of a new entity, an existing physician practice can transform into a PCMH by meeting NCQA or other accrediting body requirements. For private practices that cannot afford to make a change due to financial restrictions, hospitals and health systems, as well as ACOs and CINs, can participate in supportive roles, offering these practices the necessary infrastructure or resources to develop them. For example, Mercy Health of Northwest Ohio has developed an internal team of infrastructural support and transformation coordinators, which have helped more than 20 practices receive PCMH recognition from the NCQA to date. As hospitals and health systems continue expanding their clinically integrated networks and efforts for same, this trend is likely to continue.

CONCLUSION

Today, nearly all healthcare resources are reporting that the traditional care delivery model is unsustainable, and the way of the future is through clinical integration. The unsustainability factor does *not* mean that all providers must rush into developing or participating in an ACO or CIN. It *does* mean that providers must consider contemporary alignment within the next three to five years as the reimbursement paradigm continues to shift toward value-based models and risk-based payment models expand. The integrated delivery system, as depicted by Figure 2-6, describes the desired outcome for all providers who are contemplating contemporary alignment.

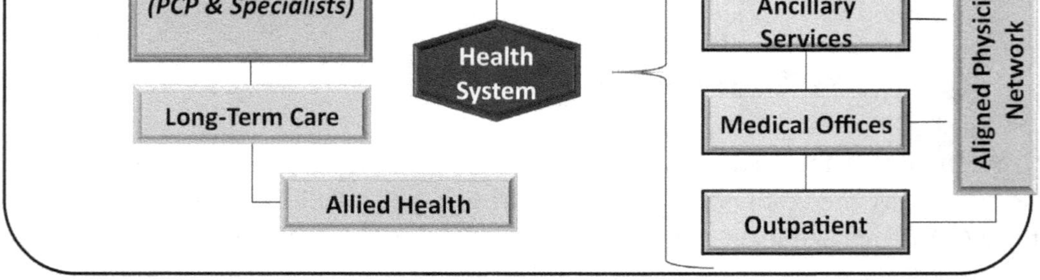

FIGURE 2-6. The Integrated Delivery System

Regardless of the pathway taken or the model chosen, the ultimate goal for progressive providers is to establish a value-centric organization that delivers quality care at cost-effective rates to a designated group of patients through collaboration with like-minded entities.

References

1. Premier, Inc., "Accountable Care Organization and Population Health Management Trends." December 2013. https://www.premierinc.com/hospital-c-suite-survey-projects-aco-participation-double-2014. Accessed September 30, 2014.

2. Mancino, Douglas M., Tax exempt issues for accountable care organizations, *ABA Health eSource*. September 2011. 8(1), http://www.americanbar.org/newsletter/publications/aba_health_esource_home/aba_health_law_esource_1109_mancino.html. Accessed July 4, 2014.

CHAPTER 3

Alignment—Risks and Rewards

There are a number of options for alignment; each one presents some level of potential risk and reward for the health system/hospital and physician(s) taking part in the alignment strategy. This chapter considers these risks and rewards on an overarching level, not specific to any single alignment strategy, from the health system and the physician perspective.

ALIGNMENT FROM THE HEALTH SYSTEM PERSPECTIVE

Undoubtedly, alignment involves a certain degree of risk for health systems, but despite such risks, the need for alignment still exists. Health systems are willing to take on these risks to reap the resultant rewards, including baseline sustainability, increased market share, and better patient care. The following are risks and rewards health systems face when pursuing alignment strategies.

Risks

Capital Outlay

An alignment strategy often leads to the purchase of something that requires a capital outlay. It could be the purchase of a physician practice's assets, the assets of an endoscopy center, a significant piece of equipment, or simply the commitment to spend funds to further the business efforts of an entity that is the target of the alignment. Thus, from a planning perspective, alignment strategies must be factored into the health system's capital budget. In some cases, the organization's ability to pursue alignment strategies is hindered by its health and the concomitant inability to access capital.

In addition, any time capital spending is in play, a health system is focused on the return on investment of their spending. In other words, are they going to realize the necessary benefit to justify the capital expenditure? In most cases, the return on investment is perceived to be simply a monetary calculation, but in the healthcare environment, this could be viewed in more of a qualitative fashion as well. For example, when aligning with a primary care practice, the return on investment may be better access to patient care rather than the primary care practice making money for the health system.

With the varying alignment alternatives in today's environment, and physician practices literally lining up at health systems' doors looking for some sort of affiliation, the health system must weigh the risks of the capital involved in each transaction to ensure that the alignment strategy provides long-term benefit while meeting all of the necessary legal parameters.

Increased Costs

In addition to the initial capital outlay, many alignment strategies increase the ongoing costs for the health system. For example, if a health system historically has not provided compensation to physicians for call coverage, but begins to as part of the alignment strategy, costs increase for the organization. This increase can become substantial. For example, if a health system begins paying general surgery $1,000 per night for call coverage, this translates to an increased cost of $365,000 per year. Multiply this by the other specialties who will desire similar compensation, and the cost of this alignment strategy grows exponentially overnight.

The most common alignment strategy today, physician employment, entails significant added costs as well. In most cases, health systems lose money when they employ physicians because of the economics of the practice and the fact that employed physicians often see slightly higher compensation arrangements than when they were in private practice. Further, if a health system is not adept at managing physician practices, the losses tend to grow with every physician added. In addition, revenues that were previously part of the practice operations for ancillary services may be pulled out by the health system and redirected to another facility. The allocation change has a negative impact on the practice's future revenues, so the losses in revenue appear larger. Thus, while the employment of physicians may provide some benefit in meeting the health system's patient care and other goals, it may create an economically unsustainable environment.

Changing Reimbursement Environment

Another key risk that health systems take on with respect to alignment is the risk of the changing reimbursement environment. Because many physicians are paid in employed/aligned settings, they do not take on direct payer risk. While their pay may ultimately flex based on changes in the payer environment, this is by no means immediate, as it would be in private practice. Thus, in an aligned environment, health systems take on all of this risk.

In addition, many alignment strategies have been fueled based on the ability of hospitals to generate higher revenues if they "own" the ancillary asset. This has been the case for endoscopy centers, cardiology diagnostic testing, and many others. Thus, if the ability for the hospital to generate these higher revenues were to disappear, it would threaten the economics of many of the existing alignment strategies.

Concentrated Risk on Single-Provider Groups

Another consideration is the concentrated risk for single-provider groups. When many private practices provide services to a health system, there is less risk because, for example, there may be 10 different cardiologists in four separate private practices providing services. As employment grows, all of those physicians are concentrated in a single provider group. Thus, if something upsets the status quo and all of the cardiologists leave, the health system risks having no cardiologists to care for patients. The principle holds true for all specialties.

Difficulty Unwinding

Another key risk health systems face with respect to alignment strategies are the unwind options if the relationship does not work out. It may not be easy for the health system to unwind the arrangement and pursue other alternatives. For example, a call pay arrangement typically is easy to unwind with a 30- to 60-day without-cause termination provision, but the employment of a large physician group is much more complicated to unwind, especially after their operations have become intertwined into the health system.

Another key issue is precedent. Using call compensation as an example, once the physicians receive payment for this service, it may be impossible to revert to an arrangement whereby physicians provide uncompensated services. The pursuit of an alternative alignment strategy often is necessary, and typically entails more risk due to the level of alignment. Therefore, regardless of the complexity of the alignment strategy, health systems must realize the unlikelihood of being able to unwind completely; some form of alignment will be the new normal for the foreseeable future.

Challenging Provider Relationships/Cultural Development

As health systems and physicians have become more aligned, the lack of cultural development/integration has become an area of focus. Many health systems have done well to develop a critical mass of aligned physicians, but few have been able to truly integrate those physicians into the overall organizations and create a collaborative culture and governance model that brings the physicians into the decision-making realm. Physicians who spent many years in private practice feel disenfranchised with their lack of ability to effect change. Additionally, the slow-moving nature of large health systems and the seemingly poor management of their practice about which the physicians can do nothing, are sources of frustration. Needless to say, this model eventually will fail, or at least result in much higher costs and less value-added than the initial vision that was cast.

Thus, developing critical mass is not enough; if a health system cannot create an effective governance model and culture wherein the physicians can thrive, not just economically, the alignment strategy is at risk of failing.

Rewards

Alignment strategies for health systems clearly entail significant risk, but they would not be pursued if there were not benefits. The following outlines key rewards of alignment strategies.

Stable Volume/Revenues

Although reimbursement in today's healthcare environment is anything but stable, pursuing alignment strategies helps ensure stability, at least from a volume perspective. As an example, a hospital that pursues an alignment relationship with local orthopedic surgeons cannot require the surgeons to refer to their facilities (without certain caveats) and clearly cannot compensate for such referrals, but undoubtedly will receive the majority of their business. This stabilizes the volume in this key area. The same is true for many other hospital-based specialties as well as primary care specialties. While the ambulatory primary care physicians do not perform any work in the hospital, they are the primary source for many of the admissions, and pursuing an alignment strategy with them helps stabilize the volume and revenue of the health system.

Ability to Negotiate with Payers

Another key benefit from alignment is in the negotiation clout with payers. As we have seen in recent cases, such as Saltzer and St. Luke's in Idaho, this clout can be perceived to be too great and detrimental to competition.[1] However, these situations are the exception and not the norm (at least currently). In most instances, health systems benefit by being able to better negotiate with payers when they are aligned with a strong physician base.

Further, as is important in today's market, these alignment strategies give a health system the ability to offer comprehensive packages of services to payers, allowing alternative payment models to be crafted or pursued. In a fragmented market that has many players, creating alternative payment models may be difficult or impossible to achieve.

Population Health Management

The benefit of better negotiations leads to advantage. While the negotiating ability is clearly an economic reward, the more qualitative, but related benefit is the ability to manage overall populations of patients. In other words, the integrated health system can manage the entire life cycle of disease, which is beneficial largely in the ability to streamline the process and have data to track and monitor the quality of care being delivered at all stages. In a fragmented healthcare market comprised of multiple providers and multiple technology platforms, population health management is more challenging than when everyone is on the same team and working from the same technology platform.

Ability to Provide Key Specialties

Another area where alignment rewards health systems is in their ability to provide key specialties or services that would otherwise be unavailable. For example, a market that would benefit from having an oncologist wherein patients could receive cancer care in their community, but that does not guarantee enough business to attract a private practicing oncologist, could pursue this service from an alignment standpoint. Alignment could occur through employment or some other affiliation arrangement.

Summary of the Health Systems' Perspective

The benefits and risks discussed here are not comprehensive; rather, the intent is to outline some of the key risks and rewards that health systems face when pursuing alignment strategies. In most cases, the rewards can far outweigh the risks, but this requires proper structuring of the alignment strategy and all players pursuing the strategy from a mutually beneficial/collaborative standpoint rather than simply pursuing "what is best for me."

ALIGNMENT FROM PHYSICIANS' PERSPECTIVES

Similar to health systems, physicians also face risks and rewards as they consider and pursue alignment strategies. This section details some of those key risks and rewards.

Risks

Lack of Control/Decision Making

A key risk for physicians as they pursue alignment strategies is a possible lack of control over decisions about their practice. In private practice, physicians make all of the decisions relative to their practice. As they enter into an alignment model, depending on the level of alignment, this control wanes, with the hospital taking over much of the decision-making process. The lack of input leaves the physicians vulnerable to the whims of the hospital and unable to truly control their practice and its future. This can lead to general feelings of disenfranchisement and unhappiness.

Ability to Unwind (or Lack Thereof)

Another key risk physicians face with alignment is the ability to unwind, or get out of the alignment transaction. The difficulty can manifest itself in many ways. For example, if a physician sells his practice to a health system, his historical practice operations may become intertwined extensively with the health system. If he wanted to leave and buy back his practice, it would be difficult, if not impossible. Thus, he would likely be forced to start from scratch to reestablish himself. The current economics of the healthcare environment would make this challenging, at best. Further, the physician usually signs a non-compete agreement with the hospital, so his ability to go across the street (or even to the next city down the road) may be constricted, leaving few, if any, options to continue practicing in the local market. The hospital may be willing to negotiate the non-compete to keep the physician in the market if the physician does not become affiliated with a key competitor to the health system during a defined period.

Unwinding presents economic challenges as well. In many cases, the economics (compensation) afforded under an alignment strategy are much better than in pure private practice. Thus, regardless of the start-up or transition costs involved, the physician may not be able to accept the economic realities of unwinding the transaction.

After a physician goes down the alignment path in today's healthcare market, there may be no going back.

Rewards

For physicians, a number of benefits come with alignment. We address the key benefits here.

Stable Economics

Although not always the case, many physicians pursue alignments because of economics. Their current state of practicing no longer can generate a fair market value wage, at least compared to what they made in the past. They align with the health system and benefit from the added resources of that health system, such as the ability to receive a market wage for their services and, even more than that, eliminate much of the financial risk that private practice entails.

Focus on the Practice of Medicine

In many cases, alignment allows the physicians to redirect their focus from running a business to practicing medicine, which is what they were trained to do. The majority of physicians go to school to learn to be physicians; few graduate with advanced business degrees in business. However, because most physicians have been in small private practices, they must also deal with the day-to-day operations of the business: revenue cycle management, payer contracting, filing taxes, personnel issues, accounts payable, etc. Even in a good economic environment, this can be taxing and even more so in today's healthcare environment. Thus, while physicians (should) still have a say in their operations post-alignment, the alignment strategy offloads some of the operational details onto health system employees who are trained to run physician practices.

Access to Resources

Another key reward that physicians realize through alignment is the access to resources. Large health systems have much greater resources than small physician practices. Thus, the horizons for the physician are opened in a variety of ways. Information technology is a great example. Health systems are able to afford the top-of-the-line electronic health records systems and other population health tools, whereas private practices often go for much less-expensive tools due to budgetary issues. Alignment allows physicians to tap into these better resources, improving their ability to care for patients.

Summary of Physicians' Perspective

Physicians experience key risks and rewards in pursuing alignment strategies. These risks and rewards are slightly more concentrated than those health systems enjoy, but are just as important. As in the case with health systems, if structured appropriately, the benefits of alignment can far outweigh the risks in the majority of circumstances.

CONCLUSION

Health systems and physicians must weigh the pros and cons of alliances and move forward with the best options based on individual needs and aspirations. One thing is certain: changes are necessary, regardless where the players are on the integration spectrum. Maintaining the status quo is not an option for the future.

Reference

1. Note: The FTC, together with the Idaho Attorney General, filed a complaint in federal district court seeking to block St. Luke's Health System, Ltd.'s acquisition of Idaho's largest independent, multi-specialty physician practice group, Saltzer Medical Group P.A. According to the joint complaint, the combination of St. Luke's and Saltzer would give it the market power to demand higher rates for healthcare services provided by primary care physicians (PCPs) in Nampa, Idaho and surrounding areas, ultimately leading to higher costs for healthcare consumers. The federal district court held that the acquisition violated Section 7 of the Clayton Act and the Idaho Competition Act, and ordered St. Luke's to fully divest itself of Saltzer's physicians and assets. Available at http://www.ftc.gov/enforcement/cases-proceedings/121-0069/st-lukes-health-system-ltd-saltzer-medical-group-pa. Accessed July 4, 2014.

CHAPTER 4

Resolving Common Alignment Challenges

Regardless of the alignment model under consideration, it is common for healthcare systems to face significant challenges as they attempt to align themselves more closely with physicians. High hopes and optimism can quickly turn to dismay and disillusionment when these entities join forces in an effort to face the many trials and tribulations inherent in the healthcare industry. Indeed, despite the fact that aligning and integrating doctors and hospitals more closely is one of the most common solutions put forth in discussions on how to reform the highly dysfunctional healthcare system, alignment is easier said than done.

Common challenges to a successful alignment model include physicians' claims that hospitals don't know how to manage physician practices. Reciprocal complaints by hospitals are that, once employed, physicians suddenly lose their motivation to produce, with resultant declines in practice revenues. In fact, post-alignment claims of this sort are so familiar that it is rare to see hospital–physician alignment efforts that don't suffer from these issues.

The question then becomes, why are these problems and conflicts so commonplace?

Furthermore, what are the root causes of these issues? Is there any validity to the hospital's claims that their employed physicians suddenly lose motivation or the physicians' claims that hospitals have extended themselves beyond their level of managerial competency? Finally, what can be done to avoid these seemingly inevitable post-alignment issues in order to bring hospitals and physicians together in a more viable structure over the long term?

To answer these questions, we first need to describe some of the fundamentally different ways that hospitals and physician practices operate.

DIFFERENT ROLES

Perhaps the elemental difference has to do with the basic business model for physician groups and hospitals or health systems. While both are healthcare service providers, the services they provide are fundamentally different, as are their primary customers. In fact, a common observation is that the doctor's customer is the patient, while the hospital's customer is the doctor. To a certain extent this is true, in that physicians occupy a unique role in the healthcare delivery system. Through historical precedent and statutory mandate, the medical profession has been granted the right and the responsibility of initiating all treatment orders within hospitals. There are exceptions to this rule, in that some other non-physician providers are granted privileges to admit and treat patients; however, in general, admitting and treating patients is the exclusive province of those with a medical doctor (MD) or doctor of osteopathy (DO) degree.

Many hospitals, especially those who enjoy not-for-profit status, also have a broader social mission that does not extend to their medical staffs. Many hospitals, even those that are privately owned and not official government or public entities, serve broader needs, such as the provision of emergency medical, behavioral health, and perinatal services, which are distinctly unprofitable, but provide great benefit to the community. On the other hand, physician groups, until recently, were predominantly private, for-profit entities with a deep commitment to their individual patients but with no feeling of a special obligation to serve the community at large. This discrepancy in commitment to community can cause significant friction between hospitals and physicians, especially when voluntary members of the medical staff are required to perform social mission activities on behalf of the hospital, such as emergency department call coverage without compensation.

Interestingly, alignment vehicles, including employment, may or may not resolve this conflict. Many hospitals view emergency call coverage and similar duties to be part of the employed physician's job description. The physician, however, may not understand this type of agreement unless it is explicitly spelled out in an employment contract and, even then, may not accept it unless it is covered by separate compensation above and beyond the physician's base salary.

DISPARATE APPROACHES TO BUDGETING AND FINANCING

Another major operational difference between hospitals and physician practices has to do with their approach to budgeting and capital financing. For the most part, hospitals tend to finance routine capital expenditures through excess revenues over expenses (operating income) and other investments that contribute to their net-profit margin. Large capital expenses, such as new facilities, may require the issuance of debt. And, of course, investor-owned, for-profit hospitals can also tap into the equity markets in order to fund large expenditures. Rare, however, is the physician group who returns excess profit at the end of the fiscal year to the practice. Instead, most practices funnel all excess cash flows into salary lines for the physicians and fund most of their capital expenses with short- and/or long-term debt.

This different approach to financing can also lead to antagonism between hospitals and employed physicians when profits generated through physician-performed processes or procedures are siphoned off for uses within the hospital beyond physician compensation. The common lament in these instances is that the hospital is profiting from the physician's efforts and not adequately rewarding those responsible for generating the profits.

CHANGES IN ANCILLARY SERVICES

This situation can become particularly contentious when hospitals acquire physician practices that provide multiple in-office ancillary services. The usual approach, driven by the wide disparity in pricing and reimbursements for practice-based ancillary services and hospital outpatient department services, is for the ancillaries to be "stripped" out of the physician practices, at least for accounting purposes, and placed into the hospital accounts where the higher prices can prevail. The consequences of this common accounting practice can be quite deleterious and dramatically inflame tensions between the employed physician network and the hospital employers. First, many patients turn to their physicians and complain vehemently when tests or procedures, which used to cost much less in the private physician practice, suddenly escalate in price when the physician becomes a hospital employee. The test seems to be the same, the equipment is no different, and the facility in which the testing is done hasn't changed, but now the price has jumped 5- or even 10-fold overnight!

Sticker shock can be especially problematic when the patient is enrolled in a so-called "consumer-driven" or "high-deductible" health plan. The higher price for ancillary testing or procedures must now come out of the patient's pocket, and patients sometimes become bitter about paying much more for the same healthcare services. No amount of explanation about the higher overhead expenditures incurred by hospitals can appease an angry patient who has suddenly become extremely price sensitive. And, unfortunately it is often the physician who has to bear the brunt of this anger, since the patient understandably looks to the doctor as the captain of the ship who is responsible for all aspects of the practice's operations, including setting prices.

OPERATIONAL MODALITIES

Finally, it is not unusual for employed physicians and hospital employers to disagree bitterly over the way day-to-day operations are managed within physician practices. Fundamentally, running a hospital inpatient or outpatient unit is much different than managing the operations of a physician practice. Hospitals tend to centralize corporate operations, such as human resources (HR), information technology (IT), marketing, and billing, which can make physician practices feel isolated and challenged by having to wade through several layers of bureaucracy to receive the support they once could access, literally, down the hall.

Furthermore, many aspects of providing HR, IT, or marketing services to physician practices are very different than doing the same for hospital departments. The classic complaint about replacing a broken piece of office equipment, a task previously done by the office manager with a quick trip to Best Buy™ or Office Depot™, that now takes the IT department weeks to accomplish, is not apocryphal but, unfortunately, representative of the challenges hospitals face in trying to adapt their operative policies and procedures to a much different care setting with a much different set of expectations and cultural norms.

PHYSICIAN PRACTICE BILLING

Perhaps the most glaring operational problem that occurred when hospitals first acquired physician practices was the hospital's incompetency regarding physician practice billing.

Hospitals often found the specific services and scale of physician charges and revenues for those services difficult to manage with the hospital billing systems. Physicians vehemently complained that hospitals casually wrote off large amounts of money that the billing offices in well-run physician practices would pursue with vigor. Now, most hospitals understand their shortcomings when it comes to physician practice billing. Therefore, most hospitals with significant numbers of physician employees have separate billing departments for these providers and, thus, have avoided the pitfalls of admixing hospital and physician billing. Unfortunately, lessons learned in the billing department have not been applied to other areas, such as IT. There, conflicts between hospital and physician continue.

NON-PARALLEL MISSIONS

Another major source of hospital-physician disagreement stems from the vastly different cultural norms within hospitals and physician groups. As mentioned, most hospitals do have some sense of social mission; however, while this may be an important part of the cultural makeup of a large, public, not-for-profit, academic teaching hospital, the majority of American hospitals see themselves first and foremost as businesses functioning in the segment of the larger service sector devoted to healthcare service delivery. Most physician practices, however, are very loose confederations of professionals who see the business aspect of what they do as somewhat secondary to their primary mission of patient care. Again, exceptions exist and some, especially larger physician practices, are well-run business entities. However, these may be the exceptions that prove the rule. Furthermore, while some physicians see themselves as having just as much business savvy as they do clinical acumen, the norm is for most small, two-to-three-person physician practices, which make up the vast majority of practices in most communities, to be poorly managed from a business standpoint.

This difference in culture plays out in many ways, perhaps most particularly in those physician specialties that are deemed to be of special value to hospital business managers. It is not uncommon for hospitals to vigorously pursue the employment of cardiologists and orthopedists, nor is it uncommon for hospitals to invest huge amounts of resources constructing new wings full of high-tech equipment in order to recruit and retain specialists in these highly lucrative specialties. Meanwhile, other specialists, particularly in the primary care areas, psychiatry, and even general surgery, are treated like second-class citizens and receive short shrift from the hospital hierarchy. This, of course, can lead to major resentments and become especially problematic when market dynamics change and previously ignored or poorly supported specialties like primary care suddenly become highly sought after in order to supply adequate manpower for initiatives like population health management.

Physicians are no different than others when it comes to being able to harbor resentments over long periods of time. Hospital managers would do well to remember that nothing stays the same, and the revenue centers of today can quickly become the cost centers of tomorrow. In fact, it's rarely good business to put all your eggs in one basket. Therefore, a broad-based, multi-specialty, physician employment strategy is the soundest approach.

PATIENT SATISFACTION SCORES

Another common source of disagreement between hospitals and physicians has to do with patient satisfaction scores. With the arrival of tying reimbursements to scores on satisfaction surveys, such as the Hospital Consumer Assessment of Healthcare Providers and Systems (HCAHPS) or The Clinician and Group Consumer Assessment of Healthcare Providers and Systems (CGCAHPS), hospitals have become increasingly aggressive in trying to push these ratings higher. In certain clinical areas, such as the emergency department, higher ratings are especially difficult to achieve. Therefore, physicians, who are held accountable for these scores, tend to think that hospital administrators are unappreciative of the challenges involved in achieving higher patient satisfaction and are unrealistic in their expectations.

QUALITY AND COST EFFICIENCY

Finally, perhaps one of the most significant challenges to overcome in hospital and physician relationships has to do with attempts by the hospital to engage physicians in quality and cost-efficiency initiatives and the physician's resistance to participate in these activities. Hospital demands for high performance on publically reported quality measures and acceptance of significant disruptions to practice patterns, such as adoption of electronic medical record systems, are common flashpoints between hospitals and physicians. In most cases, this has to do with a misalignment of incentives between the two groups, even if the doctors are employed. In fact, most hospitals now realize that employment does not necessarily equate to alignment or integration of employed physicians with hospital objectives.

IN SUMMARY: MAJOR CHALLENGES TO ALIGNMENT

To review, the major challenges related to hospital-physician alignment, especially through the employment model, include:

1. Physician dissatisfaction with the hospital's managerial capabilities and competencies;
2. The hospital's dissatisfaction with the frequent bottom-line employed physician practice losses and physicians' claims that these losses are related to drops in physician productivity once they become salaried hospital employees;
3. The physician's perception that post-employment declines in physician practice profitability are due to the hospital's accounting practices and its siphoning of lucrative ancillary service revenues into the hospital's coffers;
4. The physician's resentment at having to bear the brunt of patient complaints related to jumps in pricing after hospital acquisition of physician practices;
5. Physician's frustrations with the layers of bureaucracy present in most hospital organizations;
6. Long-lasting resentments by some specialties about perceived favoritism by the hospital for other specialties;

7. The hospital's inability to align incentives with their physician enterprise in order to engage them in quality and cost-efficiency initiatives;
8. Lack of alignment between hospitals and physicians regarding community service obligations and the frequent perception by physicians that the hospital uses physician services to meet these obligations but does not adequately reward the physicians for providing these services;
9. The regulatory restrictions that prevent hospitals from rewarding physicians for their referrals or downstream revenues and the feeling by some physicians that these restrictions are simply excuses the hospitals use to avoid paying their employed physicians a fair market price for their services; and
10. The hospital's emphasis on patient satisfaction scores, especially in areas such as the emergency department, where the practice environment makes high performance on satisfaction surveys especially difficult to achieve.

SOLUTIONS TO THE CHALLENGES

Now let's turn to possible solutions for these problems and outline some ways that hospitals and their employed physicians might avoid the erosion of their alignment and integration efforts.

First and foremost, clear expectations from both sides are vital. While it is not uncommon that both parties feel optimistic at the start of a relationship, such as employment of a doctor by a healthcare system, perhaps a little more clarity and a little less use of rose-colored glasses would help. Specific items that should be outlined in detail in employment agreements and clearly understood by both parties include:

1. A clear job description outlining the roles and responsibilities of the employed physician, especially those related to social mission activities performed at the behest of the hospital, such as emergency department (ED) call coverage, teaching of residents or medical students, and community outreach activities.
2. A well-structured compensation model that is easily understood by each physician and leaves no ambiguity about each component of the physician compensation and what activities and specific behaviors are required for the physician to receive these dollars.
3. A clear description of the physician's authority to make decisions regarding the daily operation of his or her practice. Does the physician retain practice management authority or will this be done by the hospital?
4. A clear description of mandatory referral requirements. NOTE: It is legal for hospitals to put these requirements into physician employment agreements as long as the following three opt-out situations are allowed. The physician would not be required to internally refer if:
    a. The patient expresses a desire to be referred outside the network;
    b. The patient's health plan does not cover an internal referral; or
    c. The physician believes and can document that the quality of care available through an outside referral is superior to the quality of care available through an internal referral.

5. Specification of any restrictive covenants, such as non-compete covenants, that would restrict the providers' practice activity if they were to leave hospital employment.
6. Expectations around physician behavior and consequences for not meeting these expectations (see below regarding physician code of conduct).

Some of the other items that both parties need to understand clearly prior to forming legal hospital–physician relationships can't necessarily be codified in contracts and should be covered in detailed discussions, with written documentation of what was discussed for future reference. Topics should include:

1. How will the financial accounting of the hospital-owned physician practice be handled? What ancillary services will be included in the practice P&L, and which line items will be booked on the hospital's accounts?
2. What quality and cost initiatives are of most importance to the hospital, and what are their expectations regarding employed physicians' participation in these initiatives? Will time spent on these activities be reimbursed and if so, how?
3. What are the hospital's plans regarding ancillary pricing once the physician practice is acquired? Will services such as imaging, nuclear stress testing, endoscopy, or lab testing suddenly jump in price once the hospital takes over? Who will be responsible for communicating this to patients and fielding any patient complaints?
4. What behavioral standards are expected of the employed physician? Ideally this should be outlined in a physician code of conduct that the physician agrees to in writing prior to employment. Furthermore, the process for addressing transgressions of this code of conduct should be clearly outlined and discussed, and, the physician should understand who has the authority and jurisdiction to enforce the code of conduct. Is it the hospital's organized medical staff, the hospital's chief medical officer or vice president for medical affairs, or the hospital's human resources department? Finally, if a physician is terminated as a hospital employee, how will this affect his or her status on the hospital's medical staff? Many physician contracts include "clean sweep" clauses that state that termination of employment also results in dismissal from the medical staff.
5. What are the applicable legal standards (Stark, Anti-Kickback, Anti-Trust) that govern the hospital's physician employment agreements and how are these statutes applicable to the physician's specific agreement with the hospital? Here it is vital that physicians understand the hospital's inability to reward them for referrals. Indeed, many physicians expect their contributions to downstream revenue to be recognized in their compensation. These physicians need to understand that this is not possible and that violations of these laws can have serious consequences for the hospital and the employed doctors.
6. An understanding of the challenges of clinical practice, particularly in certain high-stress environments, such as the emergency department (ED) or the operating room (OR). What will be the hospital's expectations in these areas regarding patient satisfaction? Will providers who work in these locations and care for an especially difficult patient population be held to the same targeted goals on patient satisfaction surveys as physicians who practice in less-challenging arenas?

7. What is the overarching vision of the hospital or healthcare system regarding the employed physician network? How does this vision fit with the hospital's long-term strategic goals? Many times the details such as those outlined above get in the way of the employed physicians understanding the big picture and overall strategic plans of the parent organization. On the flip side, hospitals and healthcare systems often enter into physician employment relationships, sometimes with large numbers of physicians, and don't really have a long-term vision or strategy for the physician network or the system in general. Identifying and filling these strategic gaps early on can avoid lots of struggles later as activity in the hospital-physician alignment space increases.

In addition to establishing clear expectations and understandings on both sides of hospital–physician alignment arrangements, the parties can take other specific actions to avoid problems down the road.

The first recommendation, as mentioned earlier, is for the hospital to develop a sound strategy around their physician-alignment activities. Until fairly recently, the hospital was considered the physician's workshop, and hospital managers and the hospital's organized medical staff operated separately with very little alignment or integration. There are some notable exceptions to this, such as the renowned clinical model systems like Mayo or Geissinger, where hospitals and physicians are aligned and integrated. Places like Mayo or the grandfather of large staff model HMOs, Kaiser Permanente, however, have had decades to develop their unique and oftentimes successful cultures. Most community hospitals and academic medical centers simply don't have the time to develop these sorts of cultures, and the demands for more alignment and integration between hospitals and physicians is growing larger every day. Therefore, alternatives to becoming a Mayo Clinic overnight need to be established and mapped out in a physician-alignment plan.

Key to creating an effective physician-alignment plan is determining the overall rationale for closer alignment. Not long ago, the rationale for most hospitals was their desire to lock-in a strong referral base, particularly from their affiliated primary care physicians. Now, the rationale has broadened and includes engaging the medical staff on quality and patient safety issues, filling specialty gaps in the medical staff, and even tapping into the growing numbers of physicians who have management degrees and can help manage clinical operations.

The next recommendation is to consider the appropriate structure for alignment. While most of the information in this chapter has been geared toward hospital–physician employment relationships, this type of alignment is not the only option for hospitals that wish to align and integrate more closely with physicians. To better understand this, let's start with some definitions.

Alignment is generally understood to focus on the legal and economic relationships between a hospital and its physicians, including contracts, compensation, revenue production, and cost control. Different types of alignment, ranging from the most simple and loose to the most complicated and tight, include:

1. Medical staff membership;
2. Professional services agreements;

3. Management services agreements;
4. Clinical integration models (hospital sponsored ACOs, CINs or PCMHs); and
5. Employment.

Integration, on the other hand, is more focused on clinical care delivery, including matters such as IT infrastructure and interfacing, care management, care process guidelines and standardization, and managed care contracting—especially for novel value-based reimbursements such as bundled payments or capitation and population health management. Theoretically, there is no reason that integration can't occur in any of the alignment vehicles listed above; however, in practice it usually is more of a focus for clinically integrated entities such as ACOs or CINs.

So, when hospitals and physicians wish to align more closely, it is wise for them to consider all options for alignment and also determine which of these options will afford them the greatest opportunity to become integrated. This decision can be aided by the graphical comparison of the various alignment and integration models shown in Figure 4–1.

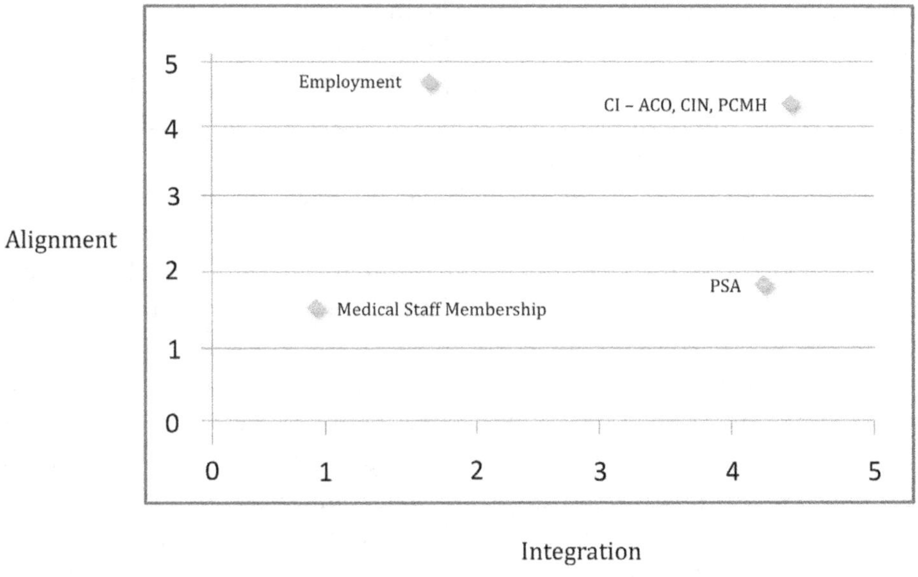

FIGURE 4–1. Alignment-Integration Spectrum

As illustrated in Figure 4–1, simple medical staff membership provides little in the way of true alignment or integration between hospitals and their medical staffs. For this reason, most hospitals are looking to other alternatives, such as developing large employed or contracted physician networks or sponsoring clinical integration programs, as a means to drive alignment and integration. Note, however, that employment does not, in and of itself, assure integration; as well, professional service agreements do not assure alignment. To maximize these two objectives, clinically integrated models such as ACOs are the most effective.

The next recommendation for avoiding and managing conflicts in hospital-physician alignment has to do with creating a sound compensation model. Several factors must be considered regardless whether the compensation is structured as salary and bonuses paid to an employed provider or a stipend is offered to an independent contractor for provision of professional services.

First, the unit of work or production must be defined. Options include a percentage of net revenues generated, net revenue minus expense, hours worked, or worked relative value units (wRVUs). The pros and cons of each are covered in Chapter 5, but it should be stated here that using revenues or revenue minus expenses as the measure of production can lead to many conflicts between hospitals, employed or contracted physicians, and other professional providers. Quite simply, using a proxy for production other than revenues, such as wRVUs, is usually the best method. Any model that measures production through the use of revenues is subject to the vagaries of managed care contracting, payer mix, and the hospital's proficiency in billing and collecting. Taking these items off the table through the use of a wRVU comp model can avoid complaints by the physicians that their level of compensation does not actually reflect the work provided and is unfairly dependent on factors outside of their control.

Finally, as the old adage says, "culture trumps strategy every time." This can be a true statement when two very different cultures like those in which hospitals and physicians have traditionally operated try to come together and form one unified culture. Hospital administrators and physicians or mid-level providers tend to look at the provision of healthcare services very differently and both carry unique historical baggage, which manifests itself in their unique, but very dissimilar, cultures.

Furthermore, the individuals within both the physician and hospital cultures bring their own unique styles and behaviors to the workplace. Meshing these into one unified culture is a complex and time-consuming process—one that cannot easily be accelerated or standardized. That being said, some recommended activities should be considered and systematically applied to the alignment process in order to expedite the blending of cultures and successful development of the desired cultural milieu.

Effective communication is probably the most important recommendation. Distrust between hospital administrators and physician/clinicians is a real problem within many organizations. This distrust stems largely from poor communication between the parties. Communicating effectively and documenting expectations, clearly articulating the vision for the future, and open, honest and transparent sharing of information can go a long way toward creating the kind of cultural cohesion that is necessary for successful alignment.

As mentioned, another element in cultural development has to do with the creation of a joint vision for the future. Indeed, this may be the most important element in building a common culture within which hospital-physician alignment can thrive. In addition, since hospitals and physicians alike are now engaged in what is perhaps the most tumultuous period of change the healthcare industry has ever known, a common vision for how healthcare reform can succeed may be the best rallying cry of all. Without a doubt, creating value, defined as quality per unit of cost, within a system that currently fails miserably at value creation, especially when compared to other healthcare systems in economically developed countries throughout the world, will succeed only if hospitals and physicians learn to set their differences aside and work together toward improving care delivery for the most important group of all, the patients they serve.

CONCLUSION

Hospital–physician alignment efforts are often unsuccessful despite the good intentions and optimism with which both parties usually enter into these agreements. Common challenges that must be overcome include a high level of distrust between the parties, different or undefined missions and visions regarding the future alignment model, failure to choose the alignment model that best meets the needs of the specific hospital and physician group entering into the agreement, and the time-intensive work that must be done to blend two very different cultures into one.

Specific recommendations for successfully maneuvering through the many challenges related to hospital-physician alignment include: clarifying the expectations of each group up-front before an alignment agreement is finalized, effectively communicating in an open and transparent fashion before and after the alignment agreement is signed, selecting the appropriate alignment vehicle that best meets the needs of the specific situation, and anticipating the unavoidable difficulties that will be encountered no matter how well intentioned both parties may be.

Perhaps the most important element in successfully navigating the treacherous shoals of hospital–physician relationships involves recognizing that no amount of carefully worded contractual language or strategic planning can overcome the cultural differences and frank distrust that exists between many hospital administrations and their medical staffs. Bringing these two cultures successfully together requires a significant commitment from both sides and a long period of time to accomplish. That being said, there is no doubt that the successful reform of a significantly flawed healthcare system depends on this cultural integration. In fact, true, long-lasting, patient-centered reform is unlikely until this comes to pass.

CHAPTER 5

Compensation Models in the Accountable Care Era

As the overall healthcare industry and, more specifically, the reimbursement environment, have changed, the incentives used to compensate physicians have also changed—or at least begun to change. This chapter explores the historical means of compensating physicians for their services and what has changed in the accountable care era. While the majority of focus will be on hospital-employed settings, due consideration also will be given to private practice settings.

HISTORY OF COMPENSATION MODELS

To better understand the current physician compensation landscape, it makes sense to first consider how physician incentives have changed over time. There has always been a strong correlation between reimbursement models and the way physicians have received compensation. This correlation is caused by the need to have a connection between what drives revenue and what drives physician compensation. While this correlation can be good for the financial performance of the organization, it also can have ulterior ramifications, such as unnecessarily driving up volume.

Figure 5-1 provides a useful picture of what compensation plans have looked like during the past several decades.

When the first wave of physician employment occurred in the 1990s, there was an altruistic sense about the arrangements. The hospitals provided the physicians guaranteed wages with the expectation that they would perform accordingly. This model failed. The fact that there was nothing other than expectations driving behavior resulted in poor financial performance, such that many health systems divested of their employment arrangements within several years after building them.

In the second wave of physician employment, health systems were smarter, offering less in terms of guaranteed pay and more compensation tied to incentive. At the time, there was very little focus on "value-based care" and, therefore, practically all of the incentive was tied to volume. The models used a variety of volume metrics, with the key metric being work-only relative value units (wRVUs). This model worked (when developed properly) in that there was a strong alignment between what drove physician compensation and what drove revenue, which at that time was predominantly, if not exclusively, fee-for-service work.

Era	Characteristics
1990s	• High guarantees • No productivity expectations • Significant benefit packages
2000s	• Strong focus on productivity (mainly wRVUs) • Guaranteed treatment largely depends on locale • Limited performance incentives (outside of productivity) • Reasonable benefit package (no more pensions)
2010s	• Continued focus on productivity, although changing • Significant focus on inclusion of performance incentives (outside of productivity) • Decreasing guarantees • Reasonable benefit package (no more pensions) • Questions of what the future looks like

FIGURE 5-1. Historical Compensation Plans

As we will discuss more in this chapter, what has transpired over the past two to three years and is still occurring is the replacement of some of the fee-for-service or volume-based incentives with value-based incentives. No longer is the sole focus on volume/revenue generation, but rather a mixture of incentives that include both volume and value.

Changes with Accountable Care

As noted, the key change with respect to compensation in the accountable care era is the shifting of incentives, and this shift is nowhere near complete. Some of the shifts have to do with the structure of physician practices. For example, historically, the healthcare industry was comprised of a number of private practices—a model that is changing dramatically. As indicated in the Merritt Hawkins 2013 Review of Physician and Advanced Practitioner Recruiting Incentives, 64% of their physician placements in 2012/2013 were for hospital employment settings, which can be compared to 11% in 2004.[1] The comparison denotes a seismic shift that has affected not only the structure of physician compensation arrangements, but also the amount of compensation being paid to physicians.

The other key change is the shift in focus of incentives. The Merritt Hawkins survey reports that 39% of their search assignments had compensation arrangements that included a quality component, as compared to only 7% in the 2011 survey.

The increase in quality considerations presents much of a challenge in the way of physician compensation. To understand why, let's look at the predominant compensation models in place today.

Historically, the "revenue-less-expense" model has always existed in private practice, wherein the revenue generated by a practice less the expenses incurred dictates the pool of compensation available for distribution to the respective physicians. This model works well when revenue is high and expenses are low, but when that is not the case, the model breaks down, as it no longer provides a market wage to the physicians. The less-than-market wage has been the case in recent years. Financial pressure on many private practices has forced them to give up their independence and to become employees of a health system so the health system can manage their practice and pay the physicians a market-based wage.

Clearly, change is happening. This change looks very different in hospital employment versus private practices. he remainder of this chapter explores specific changes that are occurring with compensation models in both the hospital employment and private practice environment.

HOSPITAL EMPLOYMENT

Much change continues to occur in the way of physician compensation in hospital-employed environments. What is interesting is that the amount of change varies substantially from health system to health system. The current physician compensation structure in place is influenced by a number of factors, which include, but are not limited to, the following:

- Overall sophistication of the health system;
- Strength of negotiating clout with payers;
- Pressure by payers in the local market to take on reimbursement risk;
- Electronic health records systems used in health systems;
- Type and number of providers employed; and
- Location of health system (urban or rural).

The compensation spectrum is broad, ranging from totally fee-for-service on one end to totally value-based on the other end, and health systems fall all across the spectrum. Some have chosen to be aggressive in their movement to value-based compensation schemes, staying ahead of the market trends. Others are taking a "wait-and-see" approach, tweaking their compensation models only after they have a firm idea of what changes are going to take hold.

Focus on Production

Several years ago, the focus of physician compensation models was almost entirely based on production. The production models, while all slightly different, have similar elements; the majority included the use of wRVUs in some manner. Even today, wRVUs are a significant element in most physician compensation arrangements.

To summarize the most basic historical compensation model, consider Figure 5-2 on the next page.

Thus, the formula has been similar, with a physician's wRVUs being multiplied by a conversion factor that translates the raw measure of productivity into cash compensa-

+ **Revenue**:
- Professional Fees (Fee-for-Service)
- ACO Income
- Call Coverage
- Third-Party Payer Initiatives
- Caption Fees
- Other

- **Overhead**:
- Direct Expenses
- Indirect Expenses
- Physician Base Salary
- Physician Benefits

= **Distributable Net Income**

FIGURE 5-2. Historical Compensation Model

tion. For example, using actual numbers, 5,000 wRVUs times a $40 conversion factor results in compensation of $200,000.

The key challenge with this model in today's environment is that the variables are limited to the extent that there is no room in the most basic formula to add in value-based incentives. Thus, the model requires substantial tweaking to be effective.

In contrast, it is worthwhile to look at another production-based model, but one that typically is exclusive to private practice: the revenue minus expenses model (Figure 5-3).

	Scenario One	Scenario Two	Scenario Three	Scenario Four
wRVUs	5,000.00	5,000.00	5,000.00	5,000.00
Conversion Factor	$40.00	$40.00	$40.00	$36.00
wRVU-Compensation	$200,000	$200,000	$200,000	$180,000
Value-Based Compensation	$0	$5,000	$20,000	$20,000
Total Compensation	$200,000	$205,000	$220,000	$200,000
Effective Comp/wRVU	$40.00	$41.00	$44.00	$40.00

FIGURE 5-3. Revenue Minus Expenses Production-Based Model

While this model can become more complex when in place, the elements are still rather simple, with all expenses incurred being subtracted from revenue, and anything left over being distributed as net income. What is interesting about this model is that it is more adaptable to the changing reimbursement environment because it can accept all types of revenue. The historical focus of this model has largely been fee-for-service revenue, yet it is just as easy to include capitation income, distributions from accountable care organizations, or other forms of value-based revenue. Thus, where a wRVU-based model is limited to fee-for-service production only, the distributable net income model can accept all forms of revenue.

The challenge with this model is that most physicians have left private practice to escape the risk that comes along with this model. Further, in hospital employment, they feel as if they have even less control over many elements of this model than they did in private practice. For example, consider that with this model, the physician:

- Has no ability to influence payer contracting;
- Is not in control of revenue cycle management;
- Cannot be payer selective (must take all patients); and
- Has limited influence over expense protocols, including:
  - Allocation of indirect expenses to the practice, and
  - Expense level of certain direct expenses (facility, personnel, etc.).

Thus, most physicians have no desire to revert to private practice-style models. What is interesting is that the model that would likely be most accommodating to the current environment is the most challenging to implement.

As we discuss production-based models, it's important to note that, in our opinion, there likely will be a continued focus on production for the foreseeable future. While some reimbursement is becoming value-based, we believe that a volume-based reimbursement will stay relevant for some time. Many health systems want to completely throw out their historical volume-based compensation models and move to a value-based arrangement. They should be cautious in doing this, as it could be problematic to have too much of a dichotomy between what is driving reimbursement and what is driving physician behavior. For example, if the reimbursement a health system is experiencing is still 90% volume-based, putting in a compensation model that is 90% value-based will misalign incentives and likely have a negative impact on financial performance. Thus, health systems must take care to ensure that there is still reasonable alignment between reimbursement and compensation models.

Focus on Value-Based Initiatives

As noted, there is a clear shift (at least beginning) from a completely volume-based compensation environment to one that includes value-based elements. Many systems are not completely throwing out their volume-based models; rather, they are supplementing them with value-based elements. This change looks different for primary care versus specialty/surgical care.

Much of the focus for primary care specialties is on population health management and accountable care activity, as these responsibilities fall on their shoulders. Therefore, this group of specialties has experienced much more change. Specifically, panel size has been inserted into compensation models to recognize the time and energy involved in managing a patient panel that is not directly reimbursed by payers. Further, significant (as a percentage of total compensation) value-based incentives are being considered, measuring how well they are doing in taking care of the respective patient panel.

Overall, specialty and surgical care has seen less activity than primary care. Still, value-based incentives are being inserted into their compensation models, but to a lesser degree of change. Further, in some instances, new reimbursement models are being considered. For example, the incidence of bundled payment arrangements for joint replacements is increasing for orthopedics. Often, the arrangement is a pilot initiative by certain payers or something that large companies in the hospital's market are pursuing in an attempt to lower the cost of care for their employees.

With respect to these value-based incentives, consider the following key elements that tend to define and drive them.

FUNDING

Funding for bundled payment incentives can come from a variety of sources, including:

- Third-party payers (Blue Cross, Aetna, United, etc.);
- Medicare (PQRS, CPCI);
- Accountable care organizations (Government or Other);
- Clinically integrated networks (CIN); and
- Internal funding.

To date, internal funding has been the largest source of funding for these incentives, but this is changing rapidly as health systems partner with various payers to address certain initiatives (e.g., PCMH) and as they become more involved in ACOs and CINs. Still, the most significant source of funding is that which the health system sets aside to pursue these initiatives.

VALUE

The value of bundled payment incentives can also vary significantly, with the following being the key factors that affect the value:

- Specialty;
- Funding source;
- Scope of incentives/measures; and
- Organizational culture.

Most health systems have started small in terms of value as they are exploring this new concept. They expand the value and scope as they become more adept at tracking, reporting, and compensating on the various metrics. The key is to place enough value wherein the physicians see a benefit from pursuing, but keep within fair market value limitations, in terms of ensuring that the scope of the metrics involved can support the value assigned. Another key consideration is rebalancing the overall economics of the model as these incentives grow. For example, consider Figure 5-4 using the wRVU compensation model example from above as a foundation.

In Scenario Two, the addition of minimal value-based incentives has a limited effect on the overall model, adding only 2.5% in additional compensation. However, Scenario Three adds an additional 10%. Scenario Four shows a rebalancing, wherein the conversion factor is reduced to make room for the value-based compensation.

FOCUS

The focus of these incentives can vary widely among organizations. Figure 5-5 depicts some of the primary focuses.

In most instances, patient satisfaction and certain quality measures are a focus within these incentives, with the other component(s) being more health system-specific. While

☒ Quality Measures	☒ Chart Completion
☒ Patient Satisfaction	☒ Administrative Adherence
☒ Expense Control (Practice)	☒ Good Citizenship
☒ Targeted Cost Savings (Hospital)	☒ Adoption of EHR
☒ Coding and Compliance	☒ Efficiency Metrics
☒ Call Coverage	☒ Medical Home

FIGURE 5-4. Compensation Scenarios

	Scenario One	Scenario Two	Scenario Three	Scenario Four
wRVUs	5,000.00	5,000.00	5,000.00	5,000.00
Conversion Factor	$40.00	$40.00	$40.00	$36.00
wRVU-Compensation	$200,000	$200,000	$200,000	$180,000
Value-Based Compensation	$0	$5,000	$20,000	$20,000
Total Compensation	$200,000	$205,000	$220,000	$200,000
Effective Comp/wRVU	$40.00	$41.00	$44.00	$40.00

FIGURE 5-5. Primary Focus Area for Incentives

patient satisfaction is somewhat straightforward, in terms of designing the incentive, quality metrics can be a bit more challenging because of the amount of data involved. Further, building certain quality measures into the incentive structure requires that they be tracked. At the onset, most health systems attempt to "piggyback" on pre-existing quality frameworks. Often, the Medicare PQRS is used as a result of the pre-established metrics that apply to many specialties. Further, many EHR systems are already set up to capture this data. Another common approach is to build the metrics currently being tracked for reporting within a participating ACO or payer initiative into the quality incentives.

Key Considerations in Value-Based Incentives

In developing the value-based incentives, certain factors should be kept in mind.

- **Development.** While the value-based incentives ultimately will represent a small portion of overall compensation, they will take more time and energy to develop than any other component. The time element is a result of the fact that value-based incentive measures are much more subjective than productivity incentives. Further, the fact that many hospitals are new to this type of incentive will require them to develop the infrastructure to support the incentives on an ongoing basis.
- **Data.** The value-based incentives are data-intensive, requiring information from many systems. Unlike a productivity incentive that relies only on the practice

management system, the value-based incentives could require information from multiple systems to support the various metrics. For example, the practice management system, hospital patient accounting system, financial system, patient satisfaction surveys, coding review reports, and others could be involved in supporting the value-based incentive structure.

Also, data accuracy is of utmost importance. The data must be tracked by the system, extracted from the system, and accurate. Otherwise, it will be difficult for physicians to buy into having a portion of their compensation tied to value-based incentives.

- **Collaboration.** It is beneficial to engage physicians in the value-based incentive process by collaborating with hospital management in terms of building the incentive structure. Collaboration will ensure that they buy into the process. In many instances, the hospital will develop a quality committee and task it with developing these incentive structures, or at least the quality incentives within the overall value-based incentive.
- **Timing of Incentive Payment.** Due to the challenges that go along with reporting on these incentives, these incentives are often paid out on an annual basis, with more frequent reporting, if possible. Once a hospital is adept at tracking and reporting on these incentives, it can consider a semi-annual payment process.

STRUCTURE

Value-based incentives can have various structures. Below are several options that are most common in today's environment.

- **Fixed Dollar Amount.** This is by far the most common structure currently in place. The hospital will simply allocate a fixed dollar amount—for example, $10,000 per physician to fund value-based incentives. The same value often applies across all specialties. Alternatively, an amount could be established for primary care ($10,000), specialty care ($15,000), and surgical care ($20,000).
- **Percentage of Base Compensation.** Another rather simplistic approach is to tie the value of the incentive to the base compensation or productivity-based compensation level. By nature, this creates some differences in the dollars assigned to the incentive based on the differing compensation levels that may exist. For example, if established at 10% of base compensation, at $150,000, this would mean $15,000; at $300,000, this would mean $30,000. At higher base compensation levels, it is important to ensure that there is enough "meat" within the incentives to justify the value assigned.
- **ACO/CIN Distributions.** Another approach is to tie any value-based incentive to distributions from any ACO, CIN, or related organization in which the hospital is participating. Thus, a physician who earned $10,000 from their performance within the organization would receive a quality incentive in that amount. The benefit to this approach is incentive to buy into the activities of the ACO, with the challenge being that the focus of the ACO may not be as all-encompassing as the hospital would desire of the value-based incentive. Further, there may be questions as to what exactly represents the physicians' portion of the ACO distribution.

The above descriptions highlight the most common structures for value-based incentives, but one of the negative aspects of these approaches is that there is no connection between the value-based incentives and performance in the productivity realm. An unproductive but high-quality physician could benefit from the value-based incentives while a physician who is highly productive but of poor quality could benefit from the productivity incentive, regardless of the performance in the non-productive realm. As a result, there has been a renewed focus on attempting to tie the productivity and value-based incentives together. One means of accomplishing this is by establishing threshold performance levels. For example, a physician must generate at least 4,500 wRVUs to participate in the value-based incentive, or the physician must meet at least 80% of the value-based criteria to achieve the full productivity incentive.

Other structures have been considered as well; each has pros and cons:

- **Variable Rate per wRVU.** In these structures, all or a portion of the rate per wRVU is tied to the achievement of value-based criteria. As an example, if the rate is set at $40, 15% of the rate is tied to value-based criteria, and the physician achieves only 50% of the value-based criteria, the ultimate rate per wRVU applied would total $37. Challenges with this approach include the fact that if base compensation is guaranteed and no productivity incentive is earned, the approach has little impact. Additionally, some physicians believe that there should not only be negative consequences for poor performance, but also incentives for high performance. One approach would be to establish the base rate per wRVU at $34 and provide the opportunity to get up to $40. Thus, it is all a matter of perspective.
- **Carve out of Base Pay.** Another approach is to carve out a portion of base compensation to tie to these incentives. For example, if base compensation is $200,000, and 15% of the base compensation is tied to these incentives, adjusted base compensation would total $170,000. The base threshold set would still be at the $200,000 level of base compensation. Thus, the physician must earn back the $30,000 of base compensation that was withheld. The main challenges associated with this approach include the fact that in order to implement, base compensation must be reduced, which is challenging in many situations. Another approach to avert having to reduce base compensation is to allow Year One's performance to impact base compensation in Year Two. Thus, at the onset, the base compensation remains unchanged and is only decreased if there is poor performance.
- **Productivity Incentive Withhold.** Another approach is to withhold a portion of a physician's earned productivity incentive and tie to these value-based incentives. As an example, if a physician earned $60,000 of productivity incentive and 25% was tied to non-productive criteria, the $45,000 would be paid out solely based on the fact that the physician was productive. The remaining amount is being withheld and paid only if the physician meets the non-productive criteria. The key challenge with this approach is that if most physicians are not earning the incentive, it has no impact.

The information, as listed, provides a high-level depiction of what is going on within health systems in the value-based realm and the key considerations being made as they continue to move further across the spectrum from a complete focus on volume/production to a more balanced focus on value-based elements. As noted, there is no single, correct strategy; health systems are developing models that work best for them based on their unique situations.

PRIVATE PRACTICE

The movement from volume to value impacts a private practice very differently than hospital employment. In hospital employment, various levers can be shifted to change the incentive structure of their employed physicians. Shifts are not so easy in private practice, considering that compensation is limited to a finite pool, with this being distributed among the physicians within the practice. Likely, there always will be a correlation between what drives revenue and what drives compensation. Otherwise, unless the practice is extremely altruistic, the economics of the practice will suffer as there will be no incentive to drive a larger compensation pool.

The inclusion of value-based incentives is difficult in a private practice when no revenue being generated is associated with such. Here, the practice has to take a portion of their revenue that was generated based completely on volume and apportion it to focus on value-based criteria. When the only factor that is affecting the generation of that revenue is volume, it is a difficult sell to tell a private practice physician he must "earn" that money twice—by doing the work and by meeting certain internally established quality criteria. Thus, it is challenging to insert value-based incentives in a private practice when it is not generating separate value-based revenue.

To overcome this, we have seen many practices pursue value-based arrangements. While some practices view this as transforming the overall focus of the practice, others see it as simply another "ancillary" service line, similar to developing a lab or imaging center. They track this revenue separately, attribute expenses to it, and then distribute any income generated from this service line to the partners of the practice or to those physicians who are participating.

In all likelihood, while these practices are initially pursuing these value-based arrangements as additional service lines, whether intended or not, as their value increases, they likely will begin to transform the practices wherein more and more of their revenue is coming from such. Therefore, it is driving behavior and, in turn, the compensation arrangement going forward.

CONCLUSION

Much is changing with respect to physician compensation arrangements, in both the hospital employment and private practice realm. As the reimbursement model continues to evolve, this change will continue, with many (if not all) health systems trying to find the right balance between volume-based and value-based incentives. As physicians are integral to the functioning of the health system and physician behavior is largely driven by what they are incentivized to do, it will be extremely important for health systems to ensure that the compensation frameworks are as effective as possible and quickly adaptable to the changing environment.

Reference

1. Merritt Hawkins' 2013 Review of Physician Recruiting Incentives. http://www.merritthawkins.com/uploadedFiles/MerrittHawkins/Pdf/2013_Review_of_Recruiting%20Incentives_Preview.pdf. Accessed July 5, 2014.

CHAPTER 6

Financial Implications in Alignment—Benefits and Concerns

After passage of the Affordable Care Act (ACA), more and more healthcare organizations are actively engaging in or working toward implementation of clinically integrated networks (CINs) and accountable care organizations (ACOs). As of January 2014, the number of entities in the Medicare shared savings ACO program is 368, up from 235 in July 2013, although about 30 have dropped out of the program in the past year.[1] The list of private sector CINs (usually involving a partnership between a private health insurer and a hospital, health system, or medical group) continues to grow. Unfortunately, some organizations are paying a steep financial price for their eagerness to curb costs, improve quality and safety, and increase patient satisfaction.

The early adopters are beginning to invest in areas such as electronic health records (EHRs), in-house case management, advanced patient-centered medical homes, and other efforts to improve the efficiency and effectiveness of the care they provide. Meanwhile, insurers in most markets are moving more slowly toward payment systems that reward the achievement of those goals. Some of the joint ventures between commercial insurers and hospitals–physician groups have produced reduced numbers of admissions, fewer total days of care, and reduced inpatient revenues across all payers, not just the payer involved in the CIN venture.

It stands to reason that the changes in practice patterns that CINs and ACOs aim to achieve will affect patients regardless of the insurer. The non-CIN insurers who have not adopted new value-based payment models are more than happy to get the free ride that comes from reduced medical utilization without having to reward the hospitals and physicians who made that reduction a reality.

BENEFICIARY PARTICIPATION

We must stress the importance of carefully modeling the potential impact a new CIN payment model may have on your patients served by an insurer you are considering for a CIN venture, and also the impact on your patients served by other insurers who are not part of the CIN. Patients' acceptance of the CIN is one of the most important factors in determining the success of these initiatives. Some patients may think that CINs are simply enhanced HMOs, and it's important that they understand the difference. Their perceptions will affect whether beneficiaries select CINs and whether they support or oppose them through political activity or other approaches. If patients view CINs as a means of making the healthcare system easier to navigate and to improve the quality of care, they are more likely to see them in a positive light. Ideally, the patients will see the CINs as a way to receive more care for their health dollars and to put critical healthcare decisions in the hands of their doctors and the hospitals in their community. [2] Patients' acceptance in turn motivates private insurers to follow the CIN model.

For hospital administrators, it is vital to clearly differentiate CINs from HMOs in their marketing efforts. Furthermore, administrators must make clear to potential patients that participation in a CIN will first and foremost increase their quality of care.

PARTICIPATION COSTS AND FINANCIAL IMPLICATIONS

An organization that wishes to form an ACO eligible to participate in Medicare's shared savings program (SSP) will face numerous challenges. The most challenging aspect of creating a CIN/ACO is the startup cost. Administrators and providers worry that the daunting costs of implementation will not be worth the seemingly low reward. Furthermore, the SSP remains incomplete, and its full implementation is questionable while many insurers, as referenced above, have taken a wait-and-see attitude. Even if the SSP does launch well and prove effective, the organization still must address the concept of forming CINs to serve commercially insured patients.

You may find that it is financially prudent to hold off on launching a CIN until you have agreements with multiple insurers, covering a sufficient proportion of your total patient population to avoid having a negative impact on your financial performance. The startup costs are a challenge with no CIN or ACO being able to predict exactly how much implementation of the entity would cost; expenditures will likely be comparable to CMS's Physician Group Practice (PGP) Demonstration. The average participating ACO in the PGP Demonstration spent $489,354 in initial costs and $1,265,897 to operate the project in the first year.[3] Consistent with those figures, CMS has estimated that most ACOs will require a $1.8 million investment to get started. However, the American Hospital Association and other organizations have estimated the average investment to be much larger.[4]

Costs are high because of the required elements and the infrastructure necessary to implement the CIN. Listed below are key elements each successful ACO/CIN must have:

- Ability to define processes to promote care quality, report on costs, and coordinate care;
- A management and leadership structure for decision making;
- A formal legal structure that allows the organization to receive and distribute bonuses to participating providers;
- The PCPs of at least 5,000 Medicare beneficiaries (required for the ACO, though the recommended size for a CIN is 5,000 or larger); and
- Contracts in place with a core group of specialist physicians.

Two major investments in setting up a CIN are 1) the organization needed to lead and manage the setup and implementation of the CIN and 2) the electronic health records (EHR). Significant leadership will be needed to structure the hierarchy of the CIN along with the reporting structures and data gathering necessary to properly report and benefit from the revenue available during this time of transition in payment models in the healthcare industry. Further, additional staff will be needed at the practice level to ensure that proper follow up is performed on all patients and the entire CIN/ACO gains the benefits of continuity of care.

ADVANTAGES OF AN ACO

The federal government is assisting in this transition under the ACA. The advantage for providers is that multiple options are available as groups that will qualify as an ACO and, since the framework is so similar, a CIN. The following are arrangements that may qualify as an ACO/CIN.[5]

- Professionals in group practice arrangements;
- Networks of individual practices of professionals;
- Partnerships or joint venture arrangements between professionals and hospitals;
- Hospitals employing professionals; and
- Other groups of providers and suppliers the secretary of the U. S. Department of Health and Human Services determines appropriate.

The variety of options available for forming an ACO presents a significant advantage. Different arrangements may work better for different providers and may be less costly to form than maintaining current arrangements.

A second advantage is Medicare's shared savings program. Essentially, the SSP gives additional reimbursement to implement a model that health organizations should be moving toward on their own. The ACO has a guarantee of at least the standard Medicare reimbursement levels for beneficiaries who require services. ACOs will face less financial risk than healthcare organizations that depend on fixed capitation payments.[6] As stated previously, the CIN framework is essentially the same, allowing you to pursue both types of reimbursement while receiving a safety net for the setup under the ACA.

Finally, the greatest advantage of CINs and ACOs, assuming they work as intended, is that they will help improve the quality of care and reduce its cost. Hospitals have the potential to be at the forefront of creating CINs and ACOs. Hospital and health system administrators should consider how embracing CINs and ACOs now will better position their organizations in the marketplace for the future.

DISADVANTAGES OF AN ACO

The proposed Centers for Medicare and Medicaid Services (CMS) rule, to appeal to consumers, incorporates a system referred to as retrospective attribution. This system will assign beneficiaries to ACOs on the basis of which physician has recently provided a plurality of the beneficiary's primary care services. Although this method will most likely be more accurate than basing attribution on the beneficiaries' overall prior use, ACOs will not know for at least the first six months of each year precisely for which beneficiaries they are accountable. While this limitation may make management of risk more difficult for the ACOs, CMS has indicated it will provide extensive data on which beneficiaries will be assigned to an ACO on the basis of previous claims.[7] For the CIN, the providers will work with the insurers to place the beneficiaries they care for under their CIN for coordination of care.

Because CMS will be basing financial benchmarks on historical per-beneficiary costs, ACOs with providers that are already efficient will have to become even more efficient.[7] This pressure, however, is slightly relieved by the fact that the yearly increase in the benchmark is a nationally uniform dollar amount per beneficiary.

The mandatory collection of quality metrics, which will have to be conducted at least partially by the ACO, could pose a significant cost to hospitals. Some of the data will come through claims; however, the ACO will have to obtain the rest through medical records or surveys. CIN quality metrics will be gathered for the commercial payers in the same manner.

Finally, CMS plans for quality measurement to evolve over the life of an ACO contract. Shifting quality metrics will place a higher perceived risk on the ACO. Providers have suggested that CMS commit to stability over the duration of a contract to help reduce the perceived risk.[7] Our expectations are that commercial payers will likewise move to shift quality metrics to higher levels, although, in the long term, the expectation is that an improved quality of care will lead to savings and benefit all parties through a shared savings allocation.

FACTORS FOR HOSPITAL ADMINISTRATORS TO CONSIDER

The shift to value-driven payment is likely unavoidable.[8] Hospital administrators have many strategic and operational factors to consider as they evaluate opportunities related to CINs and ACOs. When considering how to prepare better for CINs and ACOs, don't overlook network development. It is essential to place the right resources in the right locations to serve the target market, including care provision in the appropriate setting.[9] Fulfilling this imperative will require sufficient primary care physicians and nonphysician providers and appropriate ambulatory diagnostic and treatment facilities. Focus should also be placed on physician alignment beyond common financial incentives. For true alignment to occur, physicians must share the CIN's and ACO's vision, use agreed-upon strategies to provide evidence-based care, and employ common management practices.[9]

Hospitals can become better positioned to form a CIN and ACO by focusing on cost management. They can manage costs by reducing readmissions or shifting care to lower-cost settings, thereby eliminating unnecessary utilization, and by developing a culture focused on eliminating waste across the health system.[9] These methods will help ensure efficient use of current assets and service to the maximum number of patients.

Managing patient care also will better prepare the organization for accountable care. Hospital administrators will have to work with providers at every level of care to ensure that care management occurs across the continuum. For this approach to be effective, participants within the network must agree on best practices and incorporation of evidence-based protocols.[9]

Organizations with experience operating as an ACO or similar arrangements in providing more coordinated care to beneficiaries at a lower cost to Medicare may be perfect candidates for the Pioneer ACO Model.[10] This model allows potentially greater savings and benefits than the regular proposed SSP. The Pioneer ACO Model improves health outcomes for patients across the ACO while achieving cost savings for employers, patients, and Medicare.[10] CMS also states that the model will accommodate specific organizational and market conditions in which Pioneer ACOs work.

For organizations that are small and unprepared to form ACOs, the Advance Payment Model within the SSP may be an option. This model gives participating ACOs advance payment they will recoup later from the shared savings they earn. The Advance Payment Model is designed for small, rural, and physician-owned ACOs to assist in the initial cost of forming the ACO and participating in Medicare's SSP.[10] The Advance Payment Model would greatly benefit organizations that have the potential to save using the ACO model, but do not have the capital to cover the initial costs.

CONCLUSION

Whether an ACO is worth the high initial investment by a hospital or health system depends on the situation. Large CIN and ACO groups are more likely to benefit significantly and recover the initial costs more quickly than are small CINs and ACOs. Organizations that must make major changes in the way they provide care in order to participate may not find the program profitable initially; they will be challenged to remain viable in the future.

The pressures for accountable care are likely to increase in the future in both government-funded programs and commercial insurance. Hospitals and health systems that are not ready to enroll in Medicare's SSP initially at least should begin to make changes in the way they provide care, putting policies in place that encourage coordinated and evidence-based care and forming relationships and partnerships with other providers. This will ensure a smooth transition to a CIN and ACO when one is developed. Using the decision framework described here, hospital administrators should evaluate their organizations' capability to participate effectively in CIN and ACO initiatives.

References

1. Wyman, Oliver. ACO update: Accountable care at a tipping point. http://www.oliverwyman.com/content/dam/oliver-wyman/global/en/files/insights/health-life-sciences/2014/April/NYC-MKT08001-034%20(4).pdf. Accessed July 7, 2014.
2. Berenson, R., and Devers, K. Can accountable care organizations improve the value of health care by solving the cost and quality quandaries? Urban Institute and Robert Wood Johnson Foundation, October 2009. http://www.urban.org/uploadedpdf/411975_acountable_care_orgs.pdf. July 6, 2014.
3. Ronning, P. L. ACOs: Preparing for Medicare's shared savings program. *Healthcare Financial Management* 64(8): 46-51.
4. Reynolds, J., and D. Roble. The financial implications of ACOs for providers. *Healthcare Financial Management* 65(10): 76-82.

5. Department of Health and Human Services, Centers for Medicare & Medicaid Services (CMS). Medicare shared savings program: Accountable care organizations. *Federal Register* 76(212). http://www.gpo.gov/fdsys/pkg/FR-2011-11-02/pdf/2011-27461.pdf. Accessed July 7, 2014.
6. Correia, E. W. Accountable care organizations: The proposed regulations and the prospects for success. *Am J Manag Care* 17(8): 560-68.
7. Ginsberg, P. B. Spending to save—ACOs and the Medicare shared savings program. *N Engl J Med* 364(22): 2085-86.

CHAPTER 7

Contemporary Alignment Structures—Case Studies

As examples of the concepts of alignment set forth in the preceding chapters, this chapter describes two specific types of contemporary alignment structures. While similar in model, these two case studies demonstrate different approaches to achieving clinical integration across a diverse group of healthcare providers, including ways that physicians can take the helm of CINs.

CASE STUDY #1: PHYSICIAN-OWNED CIN

For the past 3+ years, the clinically integrated network "market" has been dominated by hospital-owned organizations. In fact, current research suggests that only 40% of ACOs are physician-owned. Despite the ownership stake, however, what is remarkable is that current literature also indicates that as many as 51% of ACOs are physician-led, and in 78% of ACOs, physicians constituted a majority of the governing board.[1] However, in recent months, physicians have begun to not only *lead* ACOs (or similar clinically integrated organizations), but also to *own* them. Specifically, hospital-owned ACOs had been the dominant (and nearly the exclusive) form of clinically integrated network (CIN) since the introduction of this concept. In recent months, however, more physicians have taken it upon themselves to form a network of providers that *own* (and thus, capitalize) a CIN and *manage* its development. While the local hospital(s) still are engaged as a contracted part of the overall enterprise, it is *physicians* who play the central role in developing the enterprise and facilitating its ongoing operations. This movement of entrepreneurial physicians engaging in their own clinically integrated activities is recent, but also represents exciting new activity within the healthcare industry, and certainly one that provides much greater opportunity for physicians to "control their own destiny" than ever before.

Case Study #1 provides a real-life example of one of the first physician-owned and led CINs (henceforth referred to as Organization A) developed in the United States. This organization developed from a 250-provider, multi-specialty IPA. It includes six specialties: ophthalmology, neurosurgery, gastroenterology, primary care (which is the major specialty to date), otolaryngology, and cardiology.

Organization A's market contains one of the largest concentrations of Medicare beneficiaries, as well as an extremely competitive Medicare Advantage environment with astonishing covered benefits. Also, this market has the third-highest uninsured rate in the nation. It is at its peak in cultural diversity. The region encompasses faith-based systems and for-profit and not-for-profit health systems. The local hospitals/systems are expanding facilities and have already begun forming clinically integrated networks (CINs) where a safety-net facility can support the significant uninsured population. In addition to a multitude of health systems, within this market is a prominent and fiercely independent physician community where the focus of integration and alignment initiatives is on IPA-development and physician-based consortiums.

As independent organizations, each private physician practice within Organization A was financially successful, able to maintain its current margins for at least another few years. The reimbursement market, while showing signs of growth in value-based payments, was still predominantly fee-for-service/fee-for-volume. The primary motivations for Organization A's IPA formation include:

- Rising consumerism and patient awareness;
- A major local health system's formation of a CIN;
- The desire to remain independent and free from alignment/integration with a hospital/health system;
- Long-term success as private practicing providers; and
- Becoming trailblazers in the value-based reimbursement space.

Although all of these were critical factors, the development of a hospital-owned CIN was a significant driver for action for the independent physicians. While not interested in developing a competing organization just for the sake of competing, the hospital-owned CIN was being developed in a manner in which the private physicians would have a diminutive voice. The fear was that the contracts, incentive payments, or shared savings that would result from their investment (through their time, adherence to protocols, attendance at meetings, etc.) in that CIN would not be nearly equal to their return. In candor, the hospital's proposed remuneration model almost assuredly resulted in a return on investment for the hospital, while it required the assumption of a significant amount of risk on the part of the physicians. (Unfortunately, this was a trend in the early years of CIN development, although this is seen much less frequently today.) Thus, the physicians, who possessed both the entrepreneurial spirit and commitment to developing their own CIN, decided to do just that.

The following events were key factors in the development of the CIN:

- Physician leadership from several participating practices met to discuss ways to attain their organizational goals without sacrificing autonomy.
- Physician leadership engaged third-party consultants to provide education on market trends and viable options for collaboration.
- Physician leadership engaged legal counsel to discuss compliance and regulatory concerns.
- The parties completed the incorporation process, leading to the development of Organization A as a legal entity.
- Physician leadership retained its consultants to create a strategic roadmap toward clinical integration.

To form an independent, integrated network of private practices to transform the clinical delivery system, the following organization goals were established and used as the drivers for all activity:

- Autonomy for individual practices/physicians within a fiscally viable network;
- Achievement of the IHI Triple Aim;
- Effective cost and outcomes measurement through an integrated IT structure;
- Alignment of CI efforts to strengthen and expand market position;
- Successful maximization of both value-based reimbursement and fee-for-service reimbursement through payer contracts; and
- Effective and strategic recruitment to strengthen the network on an ongoing basis.

To meet their goals, the physicians used a step-by-step process for developing the CIN.

Step 1. Alignment–IPA Formation: The intent first was to legally form the IPA to align each disparate group across common goals and objectives to make it more *structural* than functional and to tie each group together by *legal and economic* connections.

Step 2. Integration: The second step was to merge clinical and business models to be more *functional* than structural, tying each group together by *clinical and cultural* connections.

Step 3. Clinical Integration: The final step is intended to establish the proper IT, administrative, and operational infrastructures conducive for data sharing, and to develop a robust care delivery system that monitors, reports, and feeds back meaningful information to improve system components based on a defined set of performance measures and metrics. With this final step, the groups are tied together by *clinical and operational* connections.

Given the market competition as well as their drive to complete the transition quickly, Organization A completed Step 1 within 60 days. They then moved into Step 2 immediately thereafter, completing the Integration phase after another 120 days. Finally, they began Step 3. Organization A, as do all clinically integrated organizations (both physician and hospital-owned), learned that Step 3 is a continual process, with no real "end" date. The organization made heavy investments in a robust IT infrastructure and third-party assistance as part of Step 3, but continue to track data, monitor performance, and report to participants relative to cost and quality-based outcomes on a routine basis. This feedback loop allows for ongoing assessment and revisions to the standards and processes that are in place within the organization.

Case Study #1 Conclusions

Physician-based entities such as Organization A indicate that the control is shifting from payers to providers, and even more control is shifting from hospitals to independent physicians. Physician-based CINs can compete for risk-based contracts as much as hospital-owned CINs, and physicians are often considered the drivers of cost, so it makes sense for them to be the champions of change. Clinical integration cannot occur solely by switching financial incentives, but must include the development of a care delivery system (which is something that physicians are the most qualified to lead).

CASE STUDY #2—HOSPITAL-BASED QUALITY COLLABORATIVE

In 2009, a six-hospital, 1,250-bed not-for-profit teaching health system with a Level I Trauma Center launched its first clinically integrated quality collaborative (Organization B) including more than 500 physician participants, a data-driven large-scale CI initiative, population health management contracts with value-based reimbursements, and formalization of a horizontal management structure for key service lines (cardiac, orthopedics, women's care, neurosciences, and surgery) that supervised the patient experience and monitored and managed cost savings. Organization B was one of the first organizations in the country to pursue so many different facets of "accountable care responsive" behavior in so many different ways.

Following is a summary of the geography and market location of Organization B and the organization's efforts in each of their key markets.

Primary Market. Organization B focused on increasing efforts in care coordination alongside the major commercial payer in its primary service area. This effort resulted in the expansion of Organization B's medical home project to 3,000 covered lives after a pilot program was proven to create value. Although Organization B is in a "certificate of need state" and thus there are certain restrictions on their integration activities related to physicians, they also focused on increasing alignment efforts with the physicians in their primary market through a wide array of models (see Chapter 2 for examples of many such models).

Secondary Market. Organization B experiences fierce competition within its secondary service area, as a number of other health systems are based there. The various systems in the secondary market continue to work in competition rather than collaboration; this is exemplified in long-term legal battles over facility expansion, disputes over CON applications, and other issues. Interestingly, much like its competitors, Organization B has grown through consolidation and addition of new facilities, along with integration with its local providers. Next, Organization B has agreed to participate in a local health information exchange as a way to reduce (and hopefully, avoid) precipitous rises in costs. Finally, employers in the secondary market are increasingly using consumer-directed health plans, and Organization B has focused its efforts on targeting large employers and their readily accessible base of potential patients.

Tertiary Market. Organization B's comparatively large size has enabled it to expand its reach into its tertiary market by employing growth strategies that target physician-hospital integration. With few independent practices left (a result of physician market consolidation), it is becoming incredibly difficult for small solo practices to negotiate with payers, employers, vendors, etc. Thus, there has been a rise in seemingly unfavorable contracts from a provider perspective, which has also spurred Organization B's alignment initiatives. There is a greater prevalence of on-site clinics and value-based insurance plans because of this factor.

The first step to bring Organization B from concept to fruition was to introduce the health system's physician leaders to the concepts of clinical integration and care delivery system development as the next wave of change within the overall healthcare industry. Physician leadership then garnered the support of other physicians prior to presenting the proposal for a larger-scale CI initiative to hospital administrators. Once presented, the health system board approved funding a clinical integration initiative focused on quality and cost efficiency. The physician leadership then organized, coordinated, and oversaw the development of a clinically integrated, hospital-sponsored CIN.

Like Organization A, one of the first tasks in the planning process was to establish organizational goals. While recognizing this would be a hospital-sponsored CIN, the physician leaders wanted Organization B to remain physician-based and physician-led. As a result, they developed specific expectations for physician roles in the collaborative versus hospital roles. The hospital's role was to provide capital for developmental and CI initiatives, collaborate with physicians to maintain open channels of communication, and have the final vote on all major matters. The physicians' role was to oversee day-to-day operations of the CIN, innovate and lead novel CI initiatives, and coordinate care and develop performance measures and metrics that would steer the direction of the CIN.

In addition to remaining physician-led, the other critical goals of the CIN were 1) facilitating ongoing measurement of defined quality and cost metrics for each major specialty, 2) actively working on several large clinical integration projects, and 3) achieving success in these CI initiatives. Specifically, Organization B elected to focus their energies on four CI-related initiatives:

- Blood utilization and total knee replacement;
- Surgical supply chain standardization;
- PCMH recognition and network development; and
- Population health management for health system employees and uninsured frequent visitors to the ED.

To achieve these goals, the organization recognized the need to 1) maintain a strong IT and data system infrastructure, 2) maintain a case management/disease management/care navigator infrastructure, and 3) develop a care process design system. Across all four key initiatives, the expectation was that 1) Organization B would develop a care process design system that offers the ability to design, monitor, adjust, and produce high-value care delivery on an ongoing basis; 2) there would be a continuous care process that was data-driven with a high level of performance improvement for enhanced value to caregivers; 3) the quality and value for patients (to include the patient experience) would be enhanced; and 4) cost efficiency (eliminating waste without sacrificing quality and patient safety) would be improved, with enhanced value for the hospital-sponsor.

After the first operational year of the CIN, Organization B was able to demonstrate significant achievements. These key accomplishments include:

- $586,000 savings in blood utilization (this equates to a 7% decrease in total blood utilization costs).
- PCMH accreditation for 5 sites, with an additional 10 sites pursuing this certification.
- Orthopedic shared savings initiative that generated significant savings. These savings were split 75/25 between the sponsoring commercial payer and the CIN participants.
- OR efficiency with a $2.8M savings (this equates to 6.5% of total OR supply costs).

- Utilization of an ambulatory care team who helped ensure that 181 out of 200 patients did not experience a 30-day re-admit.

Case Study #2 Conclusions

Hospital-based CINs such as Organization B demonstrate that hospitals/health systems, which have access to greater capital, are more readily forming CINs and that these CI organizations can be hugely successful in changing both cost and quality initiatives. Nonetheless, even within a hospital-sponsored entity such as Organization B, it is critical that physicians serve as the backbone for the CIN and are the driving force for new CI initiatives. As noted above, physicians are often considered the drivers of cost, so it makes sense to make them the champions of change, *even within a hospital-sponsored model.* Ultimately, the organizations (such as Organization B) that realize physicians need to be at the forefront of discussions and planning have proven to be the most successful.

CONCLUSION

These two case studies describe how physicians can actively engage in contemporary alignment models such as clinically integrated networks. These examples have focused on hospital-based *or* physician-based entities, but it is possible to develop CINs that are jointly owned by hospitals and physicians, as opposed to the models above wherein there is a singular owner (i.e., physicians or hospital). It is likely that these models will also begin to grow in popularity when the number of successful hospital- and physician-sponsored CINs continues to increase.

CHAPTER 8

Prioritizing for the Future

As we consider the future in the context of physician alignment and related accountable care era initiatives, it is worth considering future areas of prioritization and even practical realities.

STRATEGIC IMPERATIVES

Whether or not we embrace the concepts of accountable care/physician integration/alignment, it would be a travesty for healthcare industry participants (i.e., providers, payers, etc.) not to recognize key requirements for going forward. Strategic imperatives include:

1. **Operationally sound businesses.** Every provider of healthcare—hospitals, physicians, and allied healthcare providers—must improve efficiency and effectiveness in their operational infrastructures. The improvements must apply to every facet of the business. The same principals of improved efficiency apply to clinical protocols and requirements, too.
2. **Consumer-minded "outside-the-box" delivery concepts.** Providers must embrace a new healthcare model that commits to being more patient-friendly and consumer-oriented. The concept of customer service always was important; now, in the context of future structures, it is essential.
3. **Cost controls.** We emphasize cost control throughout this book; it must continue as a major requirement going forward. Providers must become more efficient in their delivery of services to drive down the cost of delivery. Further, coordinating the care among a continuum of providers is the essence of alignment.
4. **Adjusting to change.** Whether it is the transitioning process or getting used to the new structural alignment models and/or reimbursement paradigms, providers will have to adjust and recalibrate the way they think about the delivery of healthcare in the United States.
5. **Financial incentives and structural models.** The reimbursement paradigm—the way physicians and other providers receive pay—likely will change significantly relative to methodologies for dividing up bundled payments, shared savings programs, and more. The new methods will require change management and new ways of thinking about how various actions affect an aligned group of providers.
6. **Adjusting to varying entities that will contract with payers.** The days of physicians contracting directly with commercial payers may be numbered. Now, consortiums

such as clinically integrated organizations (CIOs) will assume the role of contracting mediums for physicians and other providers—a role that will require major adjustments.

7. **Payer strategic imperatives.** Payers will have to adjust to changes that are unfolding as a result of new provider consortiums, including the following:
   - *Consumer understanding and responsiveness.* Just as providers will need a better understanding of their patients as consumers of healthcare, payers likewise will need to adjust. The adjustments include working with innovative technological advances where the patients will have more access to their healthcare-related information and will expect advances in ways to communicate and to understand their disease management and related healthcare processes. A visit to the doctor, hospital, or another healthcare provider will assume a new look in many respects. Patients will be able to see their physicians through virtual visits as technology advances and privacy and related considerations improve.
   - *Mixing business lines between government and commercial.* More than likely, the lines between government insurance-payer relations and private commercial insurance will continue to blur. As the country moves toward a modified private system (as with Medicare, Medicaid, and other government programs), payers will have to make adjustments as they work within the hybrid system.
   - *Merging provider-payer structures.* Continuing a long-term trend, many payers will initiate and develop strong provider bases within their existing delivery paradigms. Further, risk sharing reimbursement relationships will induce payers and providers to form partnerships, although they will do so reluctantly. Adjusting to new working relationships will be critical to ensure success under new reimbursement paradigms, as well as with other new accountable care era structures.
   - *Cost controls.* Now more than ever, payers also must be cognizant of controlling costs. Many see payers as having shifted the responsibility of cost controls to providers; however, going forward, it will be incumbent upon the payers to develop clinical protocols to control expenses and to limit their own administrative costs. Controlling costs will be particularly pertinent as payers operate in government segments such as Medicare Advantage programs and other newly developed structures, where the payer relationships are not entirely private (i.e., when payers operate within the government reimbursement structure).

These seven strategic imperatives will be mandatory for providers and payers to be successful within the developing and ever-changing healthcare delivery system.

A new way of thinking affects all healthcare providers. At the foundation of a new approach is the requirement to build a clinical integration strategy. Based on that strategy, providers must consider many other actions as discussed in the following section.

BUILDING A CLINICAL INTEGRATION STRATEGY

Economic pressures and healthcare reform are driving alignment between physicians and hospitals in unprecedented ways. Nevertheless, employed physicians still remain a minority for the most part, particularly for specialties outside of primary care and certain internal medicine subspecialties, such as cardiology. Unless the entity is a true "clinic model" such as the Mayo Clinic, Cleveland Clinic, or Lahey Clinic, the makeup of the medical staff–hospital relations will be a mix of employment, professional services agreements (PSAs), and private practices.

Considering the future of physician alignment in the context of healthcare reform, the most important factor will be whether the respective healthcare providers within a community (hospitals and physicians for the most part) can pull together a working relationship that is characteristic of various alignment models. The clinically integrated strategy will be the best model to respond to the accountable care era processes. At the core of this strategy are integrated systems and certain performance-based requirements. A clinically integrated organization should have the following key features:

- Overall membership of all representative providers;
- Coordinated care that is evidence-based and standardized;
- A care process design and infrastructure to respond to requirements for care coordination;
- A management system that rewards for efficiencies and overall performance;
- Incentive compensation systems that tie to performance that is not solely devoted to individual productivity;
- The ability to contract as one entity;
- Structure compliance within healthcare/CMS and antitrust/FTC parameters;

As hospitals and medical staffs consider their options, they can accept that the employed physicians are set to be in a full and complete integrated partnership with a health system. However, many, if not most physicians will not be comfortable as health system employees. The future alignment strategy, therefore, will be to find alternatives to employment, such as PSA contractual relationships.

A future alignment strategy may be the CIO/CIN structure. Many physicians now realize after they become employees or align through a contractual relationship that this was unnecessary. As second-generation contracts and resulting compensation plans unfold, many physicians are reconsidering whether to continue their working relationships. Physicians with the ability through some retained administrative infrastructure to recreate their private practice are considering such action. In fact, clinically integrated organizations that are physician owned, led, and operated are rising in prominence and appearing to be a trend.

Achieving clinical integration is not easy and will require much collaboration between hospitals and physicians. Even if physicians develop sufficient independence through a CIN/CIO, most will need to collaborate (e.g., as contractor or affiliate) with health systems in order to respond to future reimbursement requirements. Population health management will continue to be a key part of the overall structure; affiliation will be the best way for providers to respond. Those who pursue the CIN/CIO route will be responding to those needs without being employed or contracted through a professional services agreement with a hospital.

WHO WILL ADAPT BEST TO THE CHANGES GOING FORWARD?

Clinical integration is like any other major change order, both relationally and operationally. It requires significant adjustment and major acclimation, and it must be embraced by all participants to be successful. Key points to facilitate acclimation are:

1. **Create a climate for change.**
   - *Adapting quickly.* Economic pressures on both hospitals and physicians combined with new reimbursement structures should heighten a sense of urgency for adapting to a rather rapidly changing structure.
   - *Building affiliations.* Though many affiliations may be limited in their legal partnering structures, the team concepts of affiliation must exist.
   - *Capturing proper vision.* Clinical integration is not just something that is done today and declared as finished. Rather, it is an ongoing process that will continue to evolve in the coming years. Regardless of the legal definition of the structure—employment, PSA, or a more limited affiliation through a CIN—all parties must understand the purpose and work for its future success.
2. **Engage all players.**
   - *Proper and extensive communication.* Many aspects of the new vision for healthcare are difficult to understand and to accept when, for the most part, fee-for-volume/fee-for-service reimbursement still applies. The temptation is to believe that as long as the current reimbursement structure exists, the "new-fangled structures" can be ignored and deferred. For these reasons, repetitive communication about the impending changes and explanations as to their reasons is imperative. Otherwise, providers will fall short of necessary preparations.
   - *Action orientation.* With the attitude that "the sky is not falling," providers may be reluctant to act. Nevertheless, some definitive action-oriented steps and plans are important.
   - *Near-term accomplishments.* Demonstrating some "wins" will encourage those who have doubts about the value of proactive efforts and will lay the groundwork for success. Thus, it is a good strategy to the demonstrate that CIOs/CINs can produce specific carved-out shared savings or bundled payment programs, even in the midst of mostly fee-for-service reimbursement structures.
3. **Execute and continue to carry out the plan.**
   - *Future-focus.* It is important to focus on future reimbursement structures rather than exist as if the present will never end. Continued communication with some sense of timeliness and urgency are warranted.
   - *Long-term "stickiness."* Based on the belief that clinically integrated organizations are the future, no matter how soon (or how much) we develop these initiatives, we should stick to the plan of developing and maturing the CIO and not waiver. The commitment applies until such time as the market or industry changes, including healthcare reform.

FORWARD THINKING—PHYSICIAN ALIGNMENT AND HEALTHCARE REFORM

The accountable care organization regulations and, specifically, areas related to physician-hospital alignment, are still being considered in light of how best to respond from both provider and payer points of view. The proposed changes from fee-for-service to fee-for-value clearly favor those who already have significant experience managing care, managing populations, and managing risks. The requirements for tracking and maintaining cost and quality measures are challenging, yet as consortiums form, antitrust safe harbors are also undergoing challenges.

Perhaps the most incredible fact of all is that none of the accountable care era consortiums, such as Medicare, ACOs, private or commercial CINs, and other population health management entities, will work toward saving money and creating as good (or better) outcomes.

Nonetheless, the ACO/CIO requirements entail value-based purchasing, readmissions per prevention, and meaningful use requirements. These initiatives and the emphases on accountability and cost controls point to improvements in the future. Moreover, these entities will continue to exist and to be required.

What role, then, will clinical integration play in this shifting landscape? Clinical integration has been around far longer than the accountable care act, and it is regarded as a viable and necessary component of the healthcare delivery system. Its core premise is the shift from volume to value and the coordination of care. In a transparent environment, every provider takes competitive risks with the concept of value following this equation:

$$\text{Volume} = \text{Quality}/\text{Cost}$$

The justification for CIOs and ACOs increases as consensus develops on population health management outcome measurements. Recent advances in medical informatics make it easier to measure and hold providers accountable for complying with evidence-based medicine, customer satisfaction, and population management, even on a per-member-per-month basis. Medical and administrative costs are more identifiable and controllable as well.

The future of physician-hospital alignment will depend on each institution's ability to create a successful clinically integrated organization. The vision for collaboration is imperative for the hospital, physicians, or a combination of the two. The vision encompasses:

1. A network of physicians eager and willing to demonstrate a high degree of interdependence and cooperation through
2. A program of incentives designed to control costs and ensure quality, which
3. Is supported by an infrastructure that allows the physicians to evaluate and modify practice patterns.

The preferred structure to effectuate the vision for clinical integration may be a hospital network of employed physicians. However, employment is not required. Nonetheless, an infrastructure should be in place to support clinical integration and likely it will comprise both employed and private and contracted physicians. The arrangement should lead to better value for patients, providers, and employers.

CONCLUSION

The significant changes that will transpire in the near and distant future under healthcare reform compel all participants to prepare, regardless of their roles or positions. This chapter identifies imperative strategies that none of the players can afford to ignore. Those who prevail in the reformed environment are those who can adapt to the future—a future focused on alignment and integration to the degree that individual markets demand. Being forward thinking, being willing to change and adapt, and working at the highest levels of efficiencies are the prerequisites for stability and success.

CHAPTER 9

Summary

The preceding chapters address the challenges associated with alignment and focus not only on lessons learned, but also identify strategies for moving forward either to improve an existing relationship, salvage a struggling relationship, or amicably terminate a failing relationship. For those readers who have not yet aligned, these chapters provide insight into the potential roadblocks that exist and identify strategies to navigate these roadblocks, as well as develop new and different strategies aimed at success. While every potential physician alignment relationship is different, and thus, implicitly has different challenges, potential pitfalls, and definitions of success, the resources in this book aim to identify a clear pathway to a successful, balanced, compliant alignment strategy, whether you are "starting from scratch" or revising an existent strategy.

KEY THEMES

Throughout this book, several key themes for ensuring success under alignment relationships have emerged, including:

1. *Need to remain informed.* Remaining proactively educated on current trends and developments throughout the industry, as well as recognizing potential impacts to your organization within your specific market is always a key requirement to success. This education and self-awareness is vital for navigating changes and assuring fiscal and operational reliability on an ongoing basis.
2. *Need to remain nimble.* Any organization that retains unbending rigidity in its approach to alignment relationships will ultimately fail, because within healthcare, there are always opportunities to improve and change and, as noted above, different situations require different tactics and different solutions. Thus, a "one sized" approach will typically not allow for ongoing success. Rather, remaining flexible (within appropriate boundaries) is critical to success. While certainly unregulated processes and relationships are not sustainable either, there must be a balance struck between total rigidity and total leniency/variability. Remaining stagnant will never ensure success in this field.
3. *Need to recognize that there is no "perfect" alignment model.* Many people have been known to "throw in the towel" when, after the first 90 days, a newly implemented alignment structure still has some imperfections. These challenges are exceedingly normal, and for the most part, all parties need to consider the 12 month mark the threshold by which to gauge whether a relationship is on the road to success or not.

Then, even after the first year, it is critical to realize that there still may be aspects of the relationship that are not completely fine-tuned. This is also normal, and these challenges should be viewed as ongoing opportunities for assessment and improvement, rather than significant defects within the model itself.

4. *Need to recognize some alignment relationships have a (necessary) termination.* As noted above, most alignment relationships need at least 12 months to fully mature and demonstrate their value. However, after those 12 months, if there are fundamental differences that remain in philosophical approach or future outlook, it is appropriate to make an assessment as to whether the relationship is truly viable, or whether a separation is needed. Before a complete termination of the relationship is pursued, however, it is important to first look at ways to improve the relationship (as noted in #3 above). While most relationships are sufficiently vetted during the due diligence and planning process, and thus, should have the fortitude to last, this is not always the case, and it is better for the parties to recognize this and move on in different directions. Knowing when you get to that point, and then acting upon it without further tarnishing the relationship, is incredibly important.
5. *Need to develop appropriate compensation methods.* In the 1990s, when so many hospitals engaged in physician employment, one of the huge detriments to many of these types of relationships was that the established compensation arrangements were not viable. Several decades later, we need to demonstrate that we have learned from our mistakes and ensure that our current alignment relationships are built on compensation methods that will last. Otherwise, it will likely be the downfall of the entire relationship. Ensuring that the incentives (i.e., compensation) match both the goals of the parties as well as the desired outcomes of participants is critical.
6. *Need to be realistic about the anticipated financial benefits of the relationship from the outset.* All too often, parties decide to align for financially-driven motives. While there is no shame or harm in this, it is imperative that the anticipated economics (both in terms of investment and return on that investment) are well defined, clearly articulated and fully understand by all parties. For example, some physicians look at alignment as a way not only to stabilize their (often declining) incomes, but also as an opportunity to earn an additional 10—25% in income, often from the outset. If this is not a goal of their partner, this needs to be well understood as often differences in economic performance create strife between the parties and can lead to discord, or even to an unwind.
7. *Need to recognize that physician-led opportunities are increasing, and are not necessarily a bad thing.* One of the more striking developments in recent years within the healthcare industry is the increased presence of physician-driven alignment models. This is true not just from a governance perspective within a particular model, but also when considering that physicians are coming to the table with their own proposals for alignment and are truly becoming the driving force for alignment. While in the past five years we have seen many physicians approach hospitals with "hat in hand," this is changing and particularly in the last two years, more physicians are becoming proactive, visionary leaders in their own rite. While sometimes frightening for hospitals

(who often fear an ulterior motive or an impending request for financial support), this is actually a terrific advancement in the industry, and one to be embraced.

CONCLUSION

The intent of this book in the context of implementing successful accountable era initiatives is to show that there is not a "one size fits all" answer. Healthcare delivery is local and regional, with variations from locale to locale, based upon provider, public, and payer demands and preferences. It is essential to know the local and regional market and to recognize that dramatic changes can occur quickly and with little notice. Every provider should become knowledgeable in the various alignment and clinically integrated models, and they should understand where their local community's needs to expand. It is important to be aware of the changing healthcare delivery and reimbursement environment and to be alert to the risks. The best response is to recognize the needs of the locale and to react accordingly, taking action ahead of the curve. Forward thinking and good timing are fundamental for success in many ways, including and specifically developing and maintaining aligned relationships.

www.ingramcontent.com/pod-product-compliance
Lightning Source LLC
LaVergne TN
LVHW082358200926
848481LV00012B/3601
9780990724131